THE HEART OF AUTISM

Motivational Intervention Strategies for Caregivers & Professionals

by Jennifer Abeles

The Heart of Autism

Motivational Intervention Strategies for
Caregivers & Professionals

All marketing and publishing rights guaranteed to
and reserved by:

FUTURE HORIZONS INC.

721 W. Abram Street
Arlington, TX 76013

800-489-0727

817-277-0727

817-277-2270 Fax

Website: www.FHautism.com
E-mail: info@FHautism.com

© 2006 Jennifer Abeles

Cover design and text layout:
Matt Mitchell, www.mattmitchelldesign.com

ISBN: 1-932565-34-5

ISBN 13: 978-1-932565-34-8

THE AUTISM ANGEL

There is an angel who watches over us. I believe this angel is omnipresent with all of our children with autism, with all of us who need her.

She brings candor, beauty, and magic to our daily happenings. As if she knows us—she does—she guides our children to success, laughter, and joy in so many endeavors. She makes sure that Joey has this miraculous, perfect sense of balance (whew, he has so many close falls but never actually falls), Rachel finds sheer joy in playing with her Barney doll (it is happiness that I've never seen before), and Thomas eats his dried pineapples with more fervor and pleasure than a dieter sneaking a bite of cheesecake.

She is with us when we cry alone in our bedrooms, late at night, as if no one were watching. She is the one who makes sure that somehow, when we least expect it, that bonus from work comes so that we can fund hippo therapy once more—oh, how much he loves that! When we find that special, perfect fit with a teacher, a therapist, a friend—someone who truly loves caring for our child—she is behind the connection. When I hear that a magnificent, deserving child got into a prestigious, respected autism program with a waiting list a mile long, I always know who's behind it. When an exhausted mother finds a second wind and plays endlessly on the carpet of her messy living room floor with her giggling son, I turn my face upwards and smile knowingly. When I hear "you wouldn't believe me if I told you, but things went so smoothly at the doctor today," I nod my head in understanding and thanks.

The Autism Angel is behind the scenes, peeking out from behind the curtain of life and sneaking that last quick fix of our crooked costume of faith, our botched lines of courage, our stage fright from moving forward. How easy it is to forget her, but how rewarding it is to remember her! Instead of going through it all alone, we've got her right there, hovering just over us, sometimes just within us, to ensure that everything will, in fact, be "okay." Long ago, you may have been told that there is no Santa Claus, no Tooth Fairy, no Easter Bunny. But if you stopped believing in, or worse, were never told about the Autism Angel, think again! She's as real as the hair on your head, and she's smiling as you take a moment to recognize her now.

You can feel her wings gently flutter when you sit in your IEP meetings and somehow manage to come out with what you wanted and needed for your child. Her gentle, healing glow is sensed and, if you're paying attention, visible when a trauma occurs with your child and then, in the wake, all is calm once again. On your child's first day at school, she's holding his hand while he enters the classroom. And when you let it go and walk towards your car after dropping him there, she's holding yours.

Yes, the Autism Angel is a very busy lady. But she doesn't mind. She's equipped with high doses of all the things she gives us when we need them: humor, delight, faith, joy, and perhaps most glaringly, a gentle tenacity to make things right for each of us.

It is in her honor and her image that I strive to model every action I take in the world of autism.

When I'm doing a good job, I can actually feel the radiance of her smile just behind my neck, just over my shoulder where she likes to hide and hover. I smile back, and keep moving forward.

I haven't stopped yet. I don't have to: I know I'm not alone.

Jennifer Abeles

DEDICATION

I have been blessed to know a precious handful of autism angels in my own life. They cannot all be listed here, but these remarkable few are living, daily proof that angels really exist— and that there will always be autism angels to guide us all. I dedicate this book to them, and to every person in the world who lives with autism or loves someone with autism, including your child, and you. You are all my heroes.

Marian Joiner, Valerie Trinklein

If you find something of value in this book, know that at some point, it was most likely sparked, taught, or illustrated by one of these two extraordinary women and exemplary autism professionals. If you read something you don't like, they probably had nothing to do with it! Because they once saw something in me and gave me the opportunity to experience, learn, and develop professionally at their sides, they gave me the ability to see something inside every individual with autism. Marian has been my mentor. Valerie has been my role model. They are the very first true autism angels in my life.

Kayla, Nelson Atkins, Tyler Harrell

Kayla was the first child with autism who Marian brought me to meet. Her art, her heart, and her immediate openness to me astonished and inspired me. Nelson is the first child with autism I ever worked with, ever championed, and ever fell in love with. I will always cherish him. Tyler was like a beloved little brother to me who just happened to be my student. His gentle tenacity, sweet sensitivity, and unparalleled love nestled into my heart years ago and have never left. When I work with any child, I carry the vibrant memory of these three teachers and inspirations with me.

Margie, Martin, and Justin Truax

Unbeknownst to them, these three angels opened the door to autism for me. What started as an annual family attendance at the CADEF Candlelight Ball grew into a fiery passion for making a difference in the lives of those with autism. When I decided I wanted to do this work—I mean, really *do* this work—Margie led me to Marian, and guided families to me who would later become stepping stones to the knowledge I have today. Justin will always be my special grown-up autism angel, with a sense of humor, light in his eyes, and playful spirit that could trump any person without autism!

Mark Lumpkin

My partner in everything, my best friend, and the most generous spirit I've ever known. He knew nothing of autism, but jumped into this world wings first and hasn't looked back. His natural ability to befriend children and adults with and without autism has afforded me an honest and inspiring look into the potential inside every human being to connect with autism and those who have it.

ACKNOWLEDGEMENTS

Some angels fly behind the scenes. This book would not exist without these folks.

Marian and Val, I thank you with every fiber of my being, and every grain of joy in my heart. Thank you so much for everything. Kayla, Nelson, and Tyler, it is with humble gratitude that I acknowledge not what I may have done to shape the course of your lives, but what you have done to shape the course of mine. Ros and Bob Atkins, Lisa and Russell Harrell thank you for sharing your sons with me. I hope we will all connect again. Sharyn Trucks, The Hoods, and Benjamin: you brought the presence of a living angel into my life—he even looks the part! To every student, client, participant, and the original The Model Classroom, Social Butterflies, Skills For Life, and Sociabilities crews, a most sincere thanks. You are each a permanent fixture in my heart.

Veronica Zysk—you are truly an autism angel. You reminded me that it was time to finish this book and get it out there. After years of correspondence and long-distance friendship, our face-to-face meeting sparked even more love and adoration for you than I had before! Truly, you are a gifted editor, an inspired writer, and a gracious soul. When I didn't know how to approach something about this book, you got me on track. A big, glittering thank you hug goes out to you.

Renee Feldman and Jon—you kept autism in my mind and heart even when I felt sadness thinking that perhaps it had stayed behind me in Atlanta. You kept me inspired and excited about my work, and you instantly extended your friendship, wisdom, and companionship along this autism journey that we are on.

Victoria Ulmer and Kelly Gilpin are new friends to me in the world of publishing. They have patiently added their own special touches of inspiration and support to this book's journey into being. Always open, always ready to help, you are an author's dream publishing reps!

Wayne Gilpin and Future Horizons, Inc. has prompted a newfound appreciation and gratitude for the publishing world. Wayne and FHI had the vision to see that this book is truly needed and valuable, and they are the backbone responsible for its tangible presence in your hands right now.

To my parents, Rhona and Fred Abeles, who took me to my first CADEF Candlelight ball when I was twelve years old. It was the start of something remarkable, perhaps culminating in my entire connection with autism and the creation of this book.

To those in the world of autism who do great, ethical, and effective work to improve the quality of life for our children with autism, especially including the TEACCH program of UNC/Chapel Hill. I've spent enough time in this field to notice that many of the most cherished, beloved autism professionals I know have their working origins in TEACCH, and those who do not come from a TEACCH background often convey its approach whether inadvertently or deliberately. Many of the most effective strategies and approaches we use (e.g., using visual supports, structured teaching approaches, the idea that parents can be active resources for their own children) are a part of the inner-workings of the TEACCH philosophy. By visiting www.teacch.com, you can read more about this approach straight from the source, and learn how these concepts have been successfully applied by teachers, therapists, and caregivers around the globe. TEACCH, I salute you and your work.

My most remarkable thanks goes out to two individuals who may not be seen by your eyes, but whose presence can surely be felt within the pages of this book. The great sage Gandhi and his message of love, peace, and kindness has indeed cast me in the role of a ghostwriter of sorts, delivering a timeless, universal message in a new, autism-focused context. Gandhi said, "My life is my message." May I be blessed and committed enough to make my life my message as well. The other is, of course, the (real) Autism Angel. Although she is certainly a part of me that is always within me, she is also an angel of her very own identity. She is, as the trite but true song lyric might have us consider, "the wind beneath my wings." To Gandhi and the Autism Angel: thank you.

AUTHOR'S STATEMENT

This book is intended to provide practical, spiritual, and inspirational fuel to people connected with autism. It is not a religious work. People of all religions, non-religions, belief systems, and philosophies can feel comfortable amongst these pages. The affirmations and concepts embodied here are applicable and respectful to all and exclusionary to none. In reading, you may feel free to generalize or personalize the thoughts and inspirations embodied in this book, internally changing language, terminology, and other concepts to meet your own personal system of values and beliefs.

Each one of us has been blessed with a heart and soul. This book simply feeds them.

CONTENTS

Foreword xvii

Introduction xxi

Affirmation of Strength xxv

Chapter One—Burying Myths, Embracing Truths 1
Highlighting stereotypes, myths, and misconceptions about those with
autism, and illuminating the truths that undo them
Affirmation: Honoring The Truth

Chapter Two—Stories of Hope and Joy 15
Real life examples of people, programs, and places where autism has left a
positive mark or been met with success
Affirmation: Rekindling the Joy

Chapter Three—The Difference is a Gift 27
How autism can actually be an asset and a blessing in some lives
Affirmation: Accepting the Gift

Chapter Four—Making Peace With Autism............................39
How you can live within the contradiction: working to lessen the obstacles
of autism while simultaneously accepting the autistic individual
Affirmation: Making Peace With Autism

Chapter Five—Your Chance to Shine....................................51
The 20 Key Secrets to being the most powerful, effective, and positive
presence in the life of someone with autism
Affirmation: Embracing My Role

Chapter Six—Realism Meets Inspiration 115
How to handle the rough spots and challenging realities that face us in the
world of autism
Affirmation: Rising Above Challenges

Chapter Seven—The World Around You 123
Reaping the maximum benefits of the world around you and staying
connected to life outside of autism
Affirmation: The Universal Connection

Chapter Eight—Lead to Succeed 133
How you can change the way we view autism by raising your gentle
voice of autism inspiration
Affirmation: My Voice of Hope

Chapter Nine—Autism and the Divine..................................139
How spirituality can play a role in keeping your heart full and
your worries light
Affirmation: Spirituality and Autism

FOREWORD

Everyone has inside of him a piece of good news.
The good news is that you don't know how great you can be!
How much you can love!
What you can accomplish!
And what your potential is!

Anne Frank

Quotations like this one are a source of inspiration for me when my spirit is sagging, my energy tank is running on empty, and I doubt my capabilities. What I love most about this quotation is the limitless universe of possibilities it suggests—beyond even our own thoughts and imaginations! This is the stuff that dreams are made of, and reverie feeds my soul.

Dreams of a bright, limitless future for your child with autism are intrinsic for Jennifer Abeles. This is the message that Jennifer lives and breathes every minute of every hour, every hour of every day as she lovingly works with children and adults on the spectrum. Jennifer knows well the "good news" that is within each and every one of us, and her mission on earth is to help you discover it about yourself and your child!

It was out of the immeasurable light that shines from within her that this book was born. It was out of the immeasurable light that shines within you that you are here right now, holding this book in your hands.

I'll bet you don't even recognize that light, do you? Most of us don't. We're too wrapped up in existing to remember that deep within us all is an innate ability to look at our world not only through our eyes, but through a heart that simply beams with love, acceptance, peace and serenity. Autism can do that – dull our spirit, deplete our sense of wonder and awe, dim our inner vision. *The Heart of Autism* will not only remind you of that place within yourself, but teach you to reconnect with it.

Stories of hope and inspiration abound within the autism community. But, and this is a big BUT, when your own spirit is sagging, these stories are all *somebody else's* hope, *somebody else's* inspiration, *somebody else's* way of making it through the rough spots. They do help—a little—but what we long for is our own real, useable heart fuel: a personal elixir, a spirited cosmic cocktail that provides action-oriented solutions designed for real people with real lives, and energizes us to keep going, and going, and going.

You'll find all the ingredients here to do just that. *The Heart of Autism* is simply brimming with positive energy, sparkling words, iridescent phrases and truly useable concepts that will make you literally glow from within. Jennifer's uplifting tone is contagious; you can't help but feel expansive, empowered and infused with new ideas after reading a single chapter, and Jennifer gives you nine of them! If ever a book was "heaven sent" for the autism community, it's this book.

The Heart of Autism is not just about changing behavior, improving language or teaching skills to help your child succeed, although the practical guidance this book imparts may result in those achievements for your child. This book is oh, so much more.

This is "heart smart" sustenance to help you *feel* your way through autism and approach intervention from an inspiring new perspective. Jennifer supportively teaches you to draw out your own expertise and become your child's best resource. Instead of fostering dependency on outside experts, she uses her own expertise to help you become a strong, savvy autism guide. Jennifer knows that within each of you is a natural inner wisdom, a place where the answers to all of your questions about your child reside. Rather than offer a carbon copy plan designed for the multitude for you to simply emulate, she lovingly and gently guides you to awaken your own source of knowledge, inspiration and wonder. In doing so, you will clearly see your child's inner beauty, his inherent capabilities, and intervention will spring naturally from the inside, out.

This is a book that feeds your mind, yet resonates at a soul level; each time you open it, you will discover something new— about autism, about your child, about yourself. I've read hundreds of books on autism in my professional life as Executive Director of the Autism Society of America, then as book editor at Future Horizons, and, for the last six years, as editor of the *Autism-Asperger's Digest* magazine. Amidst a sea of practical books designed to educate us about autism spectrum disorders and stories that share experiences, this book will become your North Star. It is a brilliantly shining treasure that will become your personal guide. You will say, *"This was written for me."*

Veronica Zysk
October 2005

INTRODUCTION

Like a blinding flash of light, the idea for this book came to me quickly and powerfully. New clients kept coming to me with a decent-enough foundation of autism knowledge. They were always well-read and well-versed in the concepts that we eat, sleep, and breathe in the autism world: biomedical theories, neurological information, sensory indications, behavioral approaches, statistics, programs, and facts, facts, facts. It was 2000, and autism cases were on the rise. One day, I gave a copy of *Autism-Asperger's Digest* to the mom of a child new to my practice, a preschool child. I wanted the mom to read my article in the magazine—I was strutting my feathers a bit! I also steered her toward two other very informative articles, one on special education law, and the other, a firsthand narrative written by a woman with autism. The mother's response struck me as if the Liberty Bell had rung inside my head.

When the mom returned the next day, she was flabbergasted. She must have loved my article and was speechless to think that I could write such beautiful, eloquent prose! On second thought, no, that wasn't it. While touched by my article, a heartfelt account of a boy with autism, the mother was dumbfounded by the autistic woman's narrative. She didn't know that people with autism could develop into such complete, fulfilled, and self-competent individuals! In all her searching for information and valid guidance on how to raise her autistic child, this educated, intelligent mother had never before encountered a single positive, compelling account of how life can be for people on the autism spectrum. In all of her extensive reading, her searching for answers, she found only instructional, technical, medical, and scientific breakdowns of what autism is and how you address it. I passed along this same article to several other clients and friends. They, too, were taken by surprise to discover a joyful, capable, and satisfied human being with autism, with great talent to express herself via the written word. Feedback included everything from "I didn't know autistic people could grow up to write so well," to "She has feelings that are so real—isn't that unusual," to "She must be very, very mild, right? I mean, autistic people don't just grow up to be like that—she's gotta be one in a million or something."

I began to reflect upon the true spiritual emptiness that our current autism resources provide. Anyone who can read has access to a wealth of important knowledge and data regarding autism. But I didn't want my clients to simply learn *what* autism is. I wanted them to know *who* autism is! What good is a pile of informative facts regarding autism if you don't know they lead to something bigger, something more human? The spiritual void in these materials was contributing to a bleak, sometimes inaccurate and often very sketchy picture of life for *people* with autism. Think about that phrase: people with autism. Autism must be humanized in order to be understood. Then I thought to myself, "How can these parents push forward at the optimal speed and level of energy their children need if they don't even understand where that effort can land them?" I wondered why we are hoarding all the "good stuff" about autism, and feeding only the very dry, technical information to parents. It is absolutely crucial that parents gain advanced knowledge on all there is to know about autism. Books, the Internet, newsletters, magazines and other publications serve a very great need by delivering this information. But it is not the *only* need for parents of children with autism. The typical world is inundated with messages of spirituality, hope, and inspiration on a daily basis. How ironic that in the special needs population, a segment of the population that has a greater need than anyone, we have no resources that offer us a sense of purpose, clarity, and faith! Parents need some sense of where the road can lead if they work with the resources available to their child. They need to know, as they know other facts they read about autism, that autism is not a dead end! This, to me, is as factual and concrete as the number of people diagnosed with autism in a given year. How can a runner reach the finish line if she doesn't even know it's there? If no one has bothered to tell her where it is, what's to stop her from simply giving up or veering off to someplace less rewarding along the trail? Like a good runner, parents of autistic children need to understand that while there are opportunities to stop all along the way, many people with autism do reach a "finish line" of sorts, a place where independence and personal happiness merge. This does not mean that they are "cured" of autism. It means that they are connected to their own best potential, success, and fulfillment—a triumph to any living being! To address this truth in a work of literature devoted entirely to the true, often-positive side of autism is not misrepresentative of reality. Parents already have an overdeveloped sense of the sad, depressing, and unfulfilling futures that can await their children. With the help of doctors, therapists, and literature, a picture of a less-than-desired future exists in the mind of every parent, because our society has been so clear, so precise, in painting it. But this book is here to remind us, or even inform if that's the case, that the dreary outlook does not stand alone. Why has the other picture—the picture that exists often enough alongside its empty counterpart—been excluded from being expressed? *We cannot change how effectively we treat and respond to autism until we change the way we see autism.* This book is written to carry out that simple, yet absolutely paramount purpose: to express the comprehensive reality of autism and the people who live with it. To empower those in the most critical position to influence a child's life—parents, caregivers, teachers, professionals—to understand the motivations, the beliefs, and the systems of thought that ultimately lead to stronger, better successes for those with autism. It's designed to provide clear, decisive insight into effective intervention, actions, and stories above and beyond what is found in other resources, speaking to the very hearts of those who are on the front lines of autism intervention daily. It's a critical resource designed to help you keep your own child's "finish line" in sight. Within these pages you will find the joyful truths, the inspiring profiles, and the spiritual fuel that will help keep you moving forward towards your child's hopeful, bright future. Not every child with autism will grow up to have a typical life. In fact, very few will. As you read, you will embrace the extraordinary tales and heartfelt truths that positively impact many of our friends on the autism spectrum, and I know you'll join me in noting that they are anything but typical.

Love, Light, and Laughter,
Jennifer R. Abeles

AFFIRMATION OF STRENGTH

Please fill me daily with the strength, motivation, and energy to understand and see the hidden blessings that autism brings into my life. I am only human. There are days when I feel as though I cannot do it, when I think I cannot take it anymore. I worry for my child, I become exhausted working towards a future that I cannot see. Help me remember that YOU can see where my (child's) life is going! Give me a daily sense of renewal, bringing forth the strength, courage, and belief that truly lies within me. Fill my life with joys and precious, sacred moments when autism is not to be feared, but appreciated. Let me see the beauty, wisdom, and inner glow that lies deep within the heart of autism. Let me make peace with autism, so that I may then have peace in my life.

Give me the energy to lovingly complete another day of progress.

Give me the motivation to move steadily forward on behalf of my (child's) life.

Give me the joy to embrace my life and the lives of my family members and friends just as they are.

Remind me that, in truth, everything in my life is already in perfect, divine order right now.

CHAPTER ONE

BURYING MYTHS,

EMBRACING TRUTHS

- ❤ Highlighting stereotypes, myths, and misconceptions about those with autism, and illuminating the truths that undo them

- ❤ Affirmation: Honoring The Truth

"The pure and simple truth is rarely pure and never simple."
-Oscar Wilde

"The greatest truth must be that in every man, every child is the potential for greatness."
-Robert Kennedy

They say, "The truth shall set you free." If that's true for all of us, then it's especially powerful for our friends and loved ones with autism. Often stereotyped and locked behind old, rigid ideas about autism, those who live with the disorder in their lives have been waiting for a book like this to be written, for a chapter like this to be read. Before even beginning to connect with the helpful, positive, realistic, and meaningful truths that autism presents in our lives, we must first recognize the extreme value of releasing old beliefs about autism that no longer serve us. For every mother of a newly diagnosed child, every fresh teacher or caregiver, and every child born with autism, we must do this. When we bring the truth about autism into the light, all that is based in fear will crumble away, and those with autism are free to be understood and accepted. Most importantly, they are free to be treated effectively and appropriately for who they really are, not whom we have mistakenly labeled them to be. Releasing falsehoods about autism and its implications is the first step in empowering yourself to reap maximum potential and success along the autism journey.

Just ten years ago, it was understood that one in every ten thousand children would have an autism spectrum disorder. Fewer people were identified as having autism, and not surprisingly, fewer facts were known about autism and embraced in the public light. While many of the most rampant stereotypes began before then, running as deep into our medical and historical past as forty years ago, efforts have been insufficient at worst, and minimal at best to extinguish many outdated beliefs about autistic people. At the time of this book, an astonishing one in every 166 newborn babies will be born with a type of autism spectrum disorder. That makes autism one of the most common childhood disorders in the country! With so many children having autism, we'll soon be welcoming many, many new teens and adults with autism into our communities. And with many children and adults with autism in our communities, it's more important than ever that we begin now to undo the stereotypes, myths, and misconceptions that can be harmful and hurtful to those living with autism daily. Perhaps most significantly, dissolving inaccurate stereotypes about children and adults with autism is absolutely critical to designing effective intervention strategies for them.

The widely recognized character "Rain Man" played by talented actor Dustin Hoffman is an accurate depiction of only one way of *many* that autism can manifest in a human being's life. Some people with autism are barely detectable in society as different from you or me, participating fully in the rigors and rituals of life as we know it—they are husbands, wives, teachers, scholars, and friends. Others, whose lives are more severely impacted by the implications of autism, maintain less typical behaviors in public and struggle to function within regular societal parameters. Regardless, there are many misconceptions that, if we are to be a warm, welcoming, and diverse society, we must learn to bury and release as ancient myths. Here are some of these misconstrued, stereotypical, blanket concepts:

People with autism do not show or feel affection, and they hate to be touched.

This is absolutely false. Many people with autism may not respond to or present affection in typical, recognized ways, and still others truly don't care for the toils of affection, but we are not empowered to say that they do not *feel* affection. One glance at some of the joyful hugs and kisses I've reaped over the years in this field and this myth will be blown away forever for you! It is certainly obvious that some individuals with autism do not enjoy touch by others, and even clearer that some individuals with autism seem to care very little, if at all, about the needs of those around them. But know this and take it deep into your memory as lasting, critical wisdom: *the reality that presents in some people with autism does not necessarily represent all people with autism.*

Initially, this sounds like an obvious concept. "Of course," we want to say, "I know that not everybody with autism is exactly the same. Some people are higher functioning and some are lower functioning and some are in the middle." Okay—fair enough. So can it then be said that all lower functioning individuals with autism do not feel affection and hate to be touched? Hmmm, I see—that doesn't work. Can we rightly assume that higher functioning adults with autism are fine with being touched and show affection typically? Well, oops, that's not accurate, either. And what can we say about those individuals in the moderate range of the autism spectrum—is it accurate that they will generally tolerate more touch than the lower functioning folks, and demonstrate much less feeling than the higher functioning crowd? You see how complicated and abstract it can be to try and pin down a particular truth for any *group* of individuals with autism. This is with great reason: there are only a handful of truths that apply unanimously to the collective group of people identified as having autism, and many, many more truths that emerge on an individual, varied, and distinctly unique level of difference for an individual with autism.

What is fair and true about all autistic people is this: that to varying degrees and in varying capacities, they are impacted by neurologically based developmental differences in areas of communication, social, and sensory processing. Beyond that, I'd venture so far as to say that commonalities and links are prevalent, but never assumed. For example, more people with autism present a tendency to spin objects consistently than those without autism, so the association between spinning and autism is valid. But it is not universal! Likewise, not all people with autism hate to be touched, or do not feel affection. And because many of our friends and loved ones with autism *are* significantly impacted with a communication deficit, we cannot expect them to communicate verbally or nonverbally their personal feelings and beliefs about affection or touching. So I guess that all those years ago, when very, very little was known about autism and people who have it, it was just easier to make up an official "autism stand" on affection ourselves based on common findings. But we were a bit off, and a bit too widespread in our assessment of this! Now that decades have passed, interventions have improved, and children with autism have grown up into adults with autism, we are left with residual stereotypes that are steadily and rapidly being laid to rest. I imagine now how this stereotype sits with the autistic adults who are happily married, enjoy sharing emotional and physical affection with their partners, and have birthed children themselves. And I'm thinking of them now as I share these truths with you so that, when considering this or any other stereotype outlined here, you understand the context in which the myth was developed, and the light in which it has been dismissed as false. If we assume the children with autism do not feel affection, then we are more likely to dismiss an initial absence of affection as permanent. In fact, children with autism can learn to express, to demonstrate, even to feel that which we are willing to teach! Likewise, a child who initially cringes at your touch may one day learn to cherish it—but this is much less likely if you dismiss his resistance as a solid characteristic of autism that comes with the package. If you do nothing to help desensitize him, he may respond with no change in his interest to be touched.

People with autism do not make eye contact.

This can be a problem area, but it's not true at all that people with autism unanimously don't make eye contact. How do you think they'd get by as guest speakers, college professors, professionals, and partners in relationships without looking up?! Again, the focus is not on whether or not this is true for *some* people with autism, but rather, that it is not true for *all* people with autism. Initially, lack of eye contact may have helped you and your child's diagnostician identify his or her behaviors with autism. With proper and supportive training and education, eye contact can be introduced into the reservoir of behaviors your child will utilize for life! Some adults with autism describe feeling uncomfortable or vulnerable during extended eye contact, and others indicate that the very physical details of someone's eyes can be either mesmerizing or repelling! Undoubtedly, there are things in this world that make you uncomfortable. For some people with autism, eye contact is one of them. However, like taking out the trash, attending a boring meeting, or fixing a flat tire, eye contact—however undesirable—is still a functional capability of many people with autism.

People with autism are violent and/or dangerous.

A terrible disservice to those with autism has been done here. Sometimes, violent behavior emerges in an individual with autism as a coping mechanism to the pain, stress, or frustration she/he may feel over not being able to communicate and receive needed or desired things. Consider that if someone took away your ability to speak, write, or feel pain at a sensory level, and you wanted to communicate, you might just bang your head against the wall, too. Often, people *without* autism turn to violence when frustration is at a peak and they cannot imagine another way of expressing their needs or feelings. For many of our beloved friends with autism, maybe they were born with a set of life tools that left them frustrated from the get-go. It's a theory, not a fact—but one to consider. The fact remains that when communication needs are properly and effectively managed for someone with autism, violence is almost surely absent.

We must always remember that there is a reason—whether the immediate cause or trigger is obvious or not to staff, friends, or family at the moment—behind violence of every kind. This is true not just for people with autism, but for all of us as human beings. There is a *function* behind it, and a *root* that inspired it. Alarmingly, many people do not realize this, instead believing outdated stereotypes that allow people to assume violence just "comes with" autism in some cases, and therefore tragically, nothing is done to seek or address a cause. Proper training on preventative, effective autism education—and knowing how to meet each student or person's individual needs and when that student or adult is being challenged too much all at once—will be the best tools here. Beyond prevention, when violence occurs for any reason, there are physical and psychological techniques that may be applied to help do three key things: 1) immediately reestablish first physical, then emotional safety for the autistic individual and others in the environment, 2) calm the individual short- and long-term to eliminate potential flares again in the same day and beyond, and 3) carefully evaluate the circumstances that led to the initial violence, and "ouch-proof" the curriculum, environment, and interactions from then on to help avoid future outbursts. Most violent outbursts in autistic people can be traced to one of two fundamental issues: being deprived of something they need in their perception that is not understood and addressed outside of them, or being exposed to something that is uncomfortable, threatening, or violating in their perception that is not understood or addressed outside of them. I hope you will use this information, take it to heart, and share it with many others. Understanding that there is a root cause—whether that source is neurological, emotional, or perceptual in origin—will help relieve our world of this harmful stereotype, and help eliminate the violence that stems from it.

People with autism are retarded.

While it's true that people with autism *can* carry additional diagnoses that may include retardation, autism itself is not a form of retardation, and there are plenty of autistic people who have no intellectual impairments at all. In fact, those of us without autism in this community may humbly note that sometimes, our clients and friends with autism are brilliant minds who can run circles around us on many, many topics! It's not uncommon to find a child with autism also impacted by retardation, but it's inaccurate to qualify all people with autism as retarded.

While it's so easy to look at the daily performance of a young child with autism and assume that retardation is a part of it, sometimes the behaviors and differences noted in the child should more accurately be attributed directly to the autism itself. While it might appear as if a child does not have the intelligence to understand something, the reality could actually be that she/he is in fact highly intelligent, but is struggling to process the communication through which that information is being delivered. For example, we often accurately hear talk of "receptive language deficits" associated with this issue, but know that your child's hindered ability to take words in does not necessarily mean that she/he entirely lacks the capacity to understand those same words! Sometimes, a modified teaching approach can help students get past some of the processing challenges presented by autism, and get to the heart of understanding. Decades ago, we simply didn't know that, and children with autism were automatically thought to be retarded, and often were carted off to institutions or other residential facilities based on the belief that they could not learn enough to function. This is why it's critical that we not label all people with autism as mentally retarded. If we assume early on that a child cannot understand what we teach, then we will stop putting our best efforts into teaching it! If your child with autism is impaired beyond autism and shares additional diagnoses, perhaps including mental retardation, remember that intelligence can be a relative thing. I know plenty of grown business people who can't figure out what to do when their computer screen freezes up—and plenty of autistic children with "measured below average intellectual abilities" who would have that thing fixed in two minutes or less!

People with autism are destined to a sad life.

Nope! Did you know that there is even a movement of autistic people who are so happy with their lives just as they are that they protest the idea of finding a cure? While you may or may not share their thought-provoking and unique viewpoint, what we can all take from this is that many people with autism can simply be set up for success with the right tools, services, and resources in place. It's true that many people with autism can lead dramatically restricted, limited lives by traditional standards. Some people with autism need intensive, lifetime support for even simple daily tasks like eating and dressing. But happiness—like beauty—is in the eyes of the beholder. Rather than spending time feeling sorry for those with autism, or trying to dramatically change who they are, perhaps it would serve us best to simply support who they are. By providing solid, effective intervention that optimizes the best potential of each individual, we are empowering those with autism to lead fulfilling lives on their own terms. Finding a balance between when to emphasize fitting in, and when to push embracing who you really are is something we all deal with in our lives. For those with autism, the issue is more significant, obvious, and urgent to manage. Caring parents, caregivers, and autism professionals will work with autistic people to help them find that balance for success.

Have you gained something new to think about here, or released something old here? If this information was not new to you, then value it as reinforcement that you are on the right path—bravo! If you are learning for the first time that these things are important to think about when building perspectives on autism, then applaud yourself! No matter who you are, or where you are along your own individual journey with autism, know that this truly is a bright beginning. There is so much more to come for you, and for those you love with autism!

Chapter One

AFFIRMATION:
HONORING THE TRUTH

Today, I remember that autism is not an engulfing hole of darkness to run from, but a spiraling enigma that presents a brilliant array of possibilities. The truth is, my child with autism is a one-of-a-kind living treasure, and no label or stereotype defines him. Autism is not to be feared. It is to be understood, addressed, and honored. For no amount of change or challenge, diagnosis or difference will ever cloud my vision of who my child really is underneath it all—even in partnership with it all.

There is an inherent beauty that lies within each individual with autism. I can see that beauty today. There is an inherent light within the spirit of each individual with autism. I can see that light today. There are valuable truths about autism that impact my very own child. I can see that truth today.

CHAPTER TWO

STORIES OF HOPE AND JOY

❤ Real life examples of people, programs, and places where autism has left a positive mark or been met with success

❤ Affirmation: Rekindling the Joy

"It is only with the heart that one can see rightly; what is essential is invisible to the eye."
-Antoine de Saint Exupery

This is not just another place to read cute, uplifting personal accounts and tales of glory about children with autism. This is a reservoir of hope, a bouquet of practical joys delivered through profiles that are truly, remarkably brought here just for you. These examples are collected here specifically to help bring you clarity on what defines success for those with autism, and to illuminate the diverse and inspiring ways that success can be reached. When you are empowered with true wisdom and experience from this perspective, then you may adequately apply these truths to the benefit of your own child, student, or loved one with autism. In essence, then, this chapter is really all about you, and what you choose to do with understanding of the brighter side of autism outcomes.

As you read the profiles below, reflect upon the diversity of factors in each individual case. Consider how, for some adults, autism care and intervention was not nearly what it is today when these people were children. And yet they endured and rose to the top! Think about the obstacles and barriers put in place for each one of them—and consider how similar they are to your own child's way of being in the world. Take these experiences and make them yours—apply their inspiration to your child's life as if it was practical data given to you in a scientific manual on how to address autism. Because in all my years of working in the world of autism, there is one lesson that is never revealed enough to parents when they need it most:

The level of success for a child with autism is directly related to the level of belief we as adults have in that child's ability to grow.

Ready to give up? Don't. Consider that whatever point along the autism journey that you choose to stop at will most likely become the stopping point for your child's best growth and potential forward movement. We can't control autism. We can't control what set of circumstances your child was born with, what genetic materials composed your child's existence, what neurological manifestations have differentiated your child from the typical lot. And try as we might, we know that we cannot ultimately make a square-peg child fit into a circle-child hole. Your child's "finish line" in the world of autism is one that, to a certain extent, has already been charted on his course by genetic and neurological factors that are a part of who your child is and will always be. Accepting this is freeing, because it allows you to love your child fully and completely, and work hard to win the individual race while always remembering that the finish line is not abstract—it will one day be visible to you all.

But exactly where is that finish line? Aaaah—that is the question that brings us to our greatest spiritual, emotional, and educational challenge. How do you know when your child has truly "made it" to his or her highest peak of ability, performance, and fulfillment developmentally, emotionally, behaviorally, practically—really? The answer is this:

You must always keep your eye on the finish line, but never act as if you have reached it.

Autism is the most spectacular race in all the world, because it is only won when you ignore the finish line. Though it is there, it is best to never believe you have crossed it, because this sense of ongoing effort will constantly challenge you to bring your child to new levels of life-changing achievement. Instead of capping off your child's potential at a given point, by framing autism intervention as a lifelong race with an elusive finish, you can fuel yourself with the needed momentum to keep moving in the right direction. This philosophy—to never become complacent about a string of achievements or a burst of success—has been the common theme woven amongst the hearts and minds of the most effective, caring, and successful parents and professionals I've observed over years in the world of autism. And the greatest benefactors of such a philosophy are, in fact, the children. Here's how the race was run and the finish line *never crossed* in several inspiring cases where this very philosophy made all the difference.

Emily: An Adult With Autism

Emily Craner* is a 23-year-old woman with a bright, sparkling smile—and a personality to match! Diagnosed with PDD:NOS/autism as a preschooler, Emily's doctors painted quite a bleak picture for her parents when describing what Emily's life would be like with autism. They projected that she would have dramatically limited communication skills, no friends, and no real ability to connect with others. To date, Emily's family has lost count of the number of times those doctors have been proven wrong. Emily communicates in more ways than many of us, because beyond her beautiful, eloquent verbal communication and her nearly seamless nonverbal communication (yes, complete with lovely eye contact), she sings wherever she is invited—parties, events, celebrations—and brings great beauty into the world through her astounding voice. Emily lives in Georgia. She has a boyfriend, a part-time job, and does a good amount of volunteer work reading stories to children at a local school. She's vivacious, sparkling, and delightful—and as is evident in many of her personal characteristics and behaviors, she still has autism.

* - pseudonym used by request

Jon: An Adult With Autism

Jon Feldman hasn't missed a day of work in nine years. He reports daily to a nearby elementary school, where he joyfully performs his duty as a dishwasher for the cafeteria. The children at the school love seeing Jon each day, and his fellow staff members delight in having his friendly, playful energy as a part of their workforce. At thirty-four years of age, Jon has a functional ability to effectively communicate most of his needs and desires in brief two- or three-word phrases. When out and about running errands with Renee, his mom, Jon shops with his own hard-earned money, and will accept help from Renee to communicate his desires if needed. Like any thirty-something man, Jon has some hobbies and interests outside of work. He loves roller coasters, gambling, and sampling the cuisine of diverse restaurants for dinners that often include enlisting the company of friends. Putting an emphasis on health and maintaining his handsome looks, Jon exercises daily—but that doesn't stop him from helping out in the kitchen when mom prepares a tempting

meal at home! Happiness is the prevailing emotion that Jon
exudes, and his life is full, productive, and unique.

Connor: A Child with Asperger's Syndrome

Getting the right educational plan in place for Connor has
been a challenge this year. Nine-year-olds with Asperger's aren't
a strong presence in his particular school, and his family has
worked hard to educate and motivate the teaching staff to help
him succeed. In spite of less than ideal resources, Connor is
doing well and has been placed in a regular education classroom,
with some support for math and reading in the special education
setting. He struggles with certain behaviors, including some that
are associated with his secondary diagnosis of Tourette's
Syndrome. A bright, funny, and sensitive young man, Connor
communicates beautifully with his family, and even independently identifies when the stresses at school are about to put him on
overload—a skill that remains elusive in the lives of some adults,
with or without diagnoses! During these times, Connor responsibly calls his mom, and together, they talk through the problem,
or decide that he will need to "cool off." With help in the form of
an autism advocate/consultant, Connor's educational program
has greatly improved over the last month, and he is already
responding beautifully to the implemented changes.

The Model Classroom: A Program For Students With Autism

In 1986, there were no suitable intervention programs for
Margie's son, Justin. Born with classic autism, Justin needed

intervention and help that didn't exist to meet his needs. So parents Margie and Martin created that help for him. The Model Classroom was established in a tiny, empty house adjacent to a church school so that inclusion opportunities could be utilized. Two remarkable teachers were hired, and a small handful of other children with autism became a part of the very first class of autism students at The Model Classroom. Through the perseverance of Justin's parents, teachers, and his own hard work, Justin is now in his mid-twenties and possesses better life skills, coping abilities, and an overall quality of life than could ever have been predicted all those years ago. The Model Classroom has since expanded. It serves children along the autism spectrum through a specialized program complete with inclusion opportunities to learn alongside typical peers in a fantastic new private school setting.

Cole: A Child With Autism

Cole seemed to be a typical baby until, like many children with autism, his bubbly personality and babbling stopped seemingly overnight. When autism was diagnosed shortly thereafter, his parents knew they had to do something powerful, because no autism-specific resources existed in their small rural community. A neighboring town yielded a private special education school, but they had no prior experience with autistic students. Collaboratively, the parents and teachers worked together to learn about behavioral autism techniques and to implement effective strategies. It was an uphill battle at first. Cole screamed and cried and resisted attending his new school. Slowly, he began to respond to the new teachers, program, and surroundings. Language began to surface. Eye contact developed. Independent skills were fostered, and interaction with other children began to happen. Cole's development, once at square one, progressed steadily over the years. By age six, he was demonstrating the behaviors and attitudes of a functional little boy. By age eight, Cole was able to transition to "regular school," where he continues to succeed academically and socially while meeting the behavioral expectations of his new school. His family continues to work with him on building new goals and meeting them regularly.

Shantah: A Child With Autism

Social interaction and eye contact were never a problem for this giddy, playful five-year old little girl. Since her parents can remember, Shantah has been able to "goof off" with friends and enjoy the company of others. Her language skills are also intact, and Shantah communicates on an above-average level. Diagnosed initially with PDD:NOS (later revised to a diagnosis of High Functioning Autism), Shantah is passionate about her favorite characters: The Powderpuff Girls! She recently helped her mom decorate her room with decals, toys, and a new bedspread, all with her favorite motif. When not at school, Shantah loves beating her dad at computer games, and chasing Bogie, the family dog, around their yard. Although she has a tough time sitting still for long, this beautiful young girl doesn't mind focusing on her other current pastime, stacking Jenga blocks for hours on end. At the moment, Shantah declares that she would like to be a "mad scientist" when she grows up so that she can develop a formula to help The Powderpuff Girls "beat the bad guys!"

Michelle: A Parent of a Child With Autism

Becoming an advocate was not something Michelle Guppy had planned when considering the role of parenthood. But when her son Brandon was born with autism, advocacy quickly rose to the top of her priority list. As autism became a deeply embedded, routine part of her family's existence, Michelle discovered that beyond reaching her own son, the great strides she had helped her son take could be valuable to others on the autism journey. She began writing her thoughts, feelings, and experiences with autism and submitting them to publishers and websites to share with the other families who were dealing with autism. As her involvement grew, Michelle undertook a new project: developing the Texas Autism Advocacy website. The website includes her personal stories, links to other autism resources, and information to help families in her area reach the services they need. Now, having provided a cherished gift to the parents in her community, Michelle is able to reflect upon the origin of this outreach—the unexpected differences in the life of her unparalleled child.

The Bubel/Aiken Foundation: An Organization For People With Differences

In a sea of competition, only a select handful of gifted vocalists can claim their place on the hit television phenomenon, *American Idol.* And of those who graced its stage, perhaps none can boast the impact of superstar, affable philanthropist, Clay Aiken. Amidst record deals and celebrity social events, Clay focused his energy on Mike Bubel, a young man with autism. Clay worked personally with Mike to help develop and improve his life skills, community interaction, and other important skills. Celebrity Clay remains grounded in his passion to help children with developmental differences obtain the resources and support that are so critical to a lifetime of success. The Bubel/Aiken Foundation partners Clay with Diana Bubel, Mike's down-to-earth, North Carolina mom. The homepage of their website invites visitors to join them in pledging some special commitments of the heart to those with disabilities. It just demonstrates that being famous, busy, and sought-after worldwide does not have to overshadow what's *really* important.

AFFIRMATION: REKINDLING THE JOY

This is a new moment in my life, and I choose to use this time to rekindle the joy that my life with autism has to offer me. I remember the starting point on this journey— the doctor affirming that my child has autism. But I have already come so far since then—even in such little time! Whether moments or months or years have passed since that first step into the world of autism, I have moved forward with strength, tenacity, and I have done what needed to be done for my child. There are no regrets, only joy and celebration for the great things to come for my child!

There are hundreds, even thousands, of inspirations for me to draw from daily. Sometimes, I am inspired by the voices, stories, and triumphs of others. Sometimes, I am inspired by my own child with autism, and the miraculous ways that she/he exists within the framework of all unique life.

Each day, I choose to bring the best new ideas, strategies, and formulas for success into my child's life. Autism demands it. My love enables it. My child thrives on it. And that in itself is the greatest joy I have ever known—to be blessed with the ability to change my child's world for the better, every single day.

CHAPTER THREE

THE DIFFERENCE IS A GIFT

❤ How autism can actually be an asset and a blessing in some lives

❤ Affirmation: Accepting the Gift

"Imagination is more important that knowledge."
-Albert Einstein

Chapter Three

It's so easy to see the difficulties and challenges that our friends with autism must deal with. For some, it's an inability to speak. For others, it's an inherent sense of frustration and agitation with the world around them, such as discomfort with wearing elastic-band socks, hearing the low hum of an air conditioner, bearing the flicker of a fluorescent light. Then there are the social burdens and deficits—how to make (or even want) friends, connect with coworkers, manage socially acceptable hygiene effectively, fit in at school or work without losing the self. How to refrain from flapping the hands joyously, or letting echolalia dictate the words destined to escape your lips. Managing that ever-persistent internal dialogue probing urgently, "What's happening next? Where are we going now? Will I be able to come back to this activity? Do I have to leave? What if I don't like what's next?" Indeed, there is no need for yet another resource outlining the challenging side of autism—the harder side of autism. What we need is a light to soften the darkness.

It may at first be a challenge for you to join me in my place of "accepting the gift" of autism, as I have chosen to phrase it here. It may even sound a bit "Pollyanna-ish." For what gift is this? A gift that brings struggle, pain, uncertainty, and woes to my child's doorstep—and mine? Who would talk of autism as a gift, when surely we all know it is a curse whose only redemption lies in the delivery of a cure? I do not mock you; I do not devalue your cries for a change. Rather, I invite you to reframe your perspective on autism in a way that will greatly benefit your child.

Bring your attention less to autism as a concept, and focus more readily on the individual himself who has autism.

My concept of the "gift" is not isolated to the general concept of autism, but rather, to the great blessings and beauty that have entered our world at the hands of those who have autism, and the great beauty and value that lies within those individuals with autism. I understand, dear friend: you want desperately to feel this way, but like forgiveness for a venomous enemy, you find that it does not so easily come. That's okay—I am here with you, and I will help you now.

With my own two eyes, I've seen more beautiful art created by children and adults with autism than by any other group of people on earth. I've heard the music, read the writings, and utilized the technology brought into my life by people who have autism. I've stood in awe as a three-year-old boy with autism, who had never before heard about them, pointed to a simple statue of two people embracing—people I've always privately thought of as "un-winged angels"—and proclaimed, "Angels! ANGELS! Ms. Jennifer Angels!" This from a boy with heavy echolalia and who could barely sit still. I've listened to the tales of a harried but loving mother who explains that her autistic son has been able to detect when a woman is pregnant well before she is showing, and to tell the woman both the sex—and future name—of her soon-to-come baby. This from a boy who struggles to complete a math problem or speak. And I've cried tears for a young girl, barely verbal, who directed me verbally to sit for an impromptu portrait. This from a girl whose teachers had all but gave up on her, insisting that she would never interact with or take interest in others, never draw anything but the perseverative, repetitive sketches of her favorite Saturday morning cartoon figures.

When we look at the dimly lit side of autism, we are respecting the reality that life for those who have it bears a set of different rules. But when we look at the dimly lit side of autism to the *exclusion* of the brighter side, we are denying the very humanity and spirit that exists in each individual with autism, without exception.

No form of autism diminishes the human value, personal worth, and spiritual existence of the person experiencing autism.

On the contrary, there are those with autism who embrace it as a precious resource in their productive lives, a stepping stone to effectively reaching their highest performance potential in this world. There are adults with autism who are outraged that anyone would suggest they be "cured" of their very essence. You need not share this belief, though you may, in order to extract the wisdom, meaning, and purpose within it. People with autism are *people—with autism.* They are not "autism" itself, a villainous disease that has invaded and needs to be vaporized by a magic ray gun! There is no battle between good and evil here. There is no battle between "high functioning autistics" who resent a cure and "parents of lower functioning children" who endorse a cure! Let us simply recognize that we share something unprecedented in this inadvertent offshoot of the special needs "community"—we share autism. And if we care to make better progress, better changes, and better resources for people with autism, it's time we start *listening* to the people with autism who have something to say!

Some parents of young children with autism remain completely unaware that there are, in fact, functioning adults with autism who would actually prefer not to be cured or changed in any way. People with autism who resent a cure—and they are not a tiny fringe group, but many vocal, capable adults—don't all resent the intentions of the well-meaning, loving, and concerned parents who strive for such a cure. What is perhaps so abrasive to many about the "cure" concept is the underlying idea that if people with autism need to be cured, then they are not acceptable or fully appreciated as they already are. To honor their experiential input on this issue, you need not abandon the choice to search for a cure. Instead, take time to reflect upon, honor, and acknowledge the positive contributions in our world that would not have been brought forth without autism playing its enigmatic role. You most likely already value the teachings and knowledge of Dr. Temple Grandin, the most noted individual with autism in the world. Why stop with accepting the views of one person with autism—why not honor the truth that Dr. Grandin is not alone, and that there are many other voices alongside her who speak out about autism issues in a way that can be valuable to you? It's as simple as this:

Stop expending valuable energy on hating autism, and use your internal resources instead to focus on loving the people who have autism.

It is unlikely that the most powerful interventions will ever stem from fear or hate for autism, which is dangerously counterproductive. To the contrary, the most effective, miraculous, and powerful intervention strategies that we know of today have all stemmed out of *love* for a person or people with autism! Think about it. All of the major behavioral strategies, interventions, medical revelations, and even improvements in diagnostic criteria have all shared the same origin—someone's deep, unwavering love for a person with autism, and the belief that greater things can come for that individual with continued efforts. Although this may change someday in the future, today, every single product, program, and/or therapeutic intervention claiming to be able to "cure" your child of autism has been unsuccessful at best, and fraudulent at worst.

I believe that when we stop focusing on blaming, hating, and fearing autism itself and start living with respect and appreciation for those who have autism, we will move closer and closer to a genetic and medical understanding of how autism manifests, and therefore, how to prevent it. Great things do not come out of fear. They come out of love. Until we actively work to come from a loving place in our approach to autism intervention, we will struggle to find the missing pieces of the autism puzzle. Incidentally, those autistic individuals who protest a cure have a remarkably thought-provoking and inspiring mantra to share:

I am a person, not a puzzle.

What, then, do people with autism want to see in the way of services, programs, and resources for autism? They want the very same thing that you and I want—the best quality of life. They want appropriate, effective autism intervention. They want informed, knowledgeable professionals working with them—not condescending, presumptuous professionals who stereotype them. Since every individual with autism is different, no one, not even an adult with autism, can provide a set protocol or opinion that will definitely benefit your individual child's needs. Some believe ABA was a lifesaver for them, while others resent its drilling, intensive nature. Some define an ideal society as one in which autistic people are openly accepted exactly as they are, with all of their differences and eccentricities, while others maintain that they wish they had received more intensive help at an earlier age to learn how to manage autistic behaviors and fit in. No information from any outsider will ever preside over your own instincts about your child or student! But by listening to the voices and hearts of those who have gone before you, you may find pearls of wisdom that are not available to you in the words of your doctors, therapists, family, or friends. You may find resounding echoes of your own child's future voice, not yet released for you to hear. And by drawing wisdom from those who have already walked your child's path, you are essentially honoring the gift that they have given you and your child.

The gifts of autism are everywhere, and you can choose to accept them wherever you go and however you find them.

Because autism teaches us the remarkable blessing of finding joy in even the simplest of achievements, we are able to find the gifts of autism where other families find only an everyday event. Did your child paint a beautiful picture today? It is a gift—accept it. Did he throw you a sparkling smile? It is a gift—accept it. Did your daughter take turns with your neighbor's little girl on the swing set? It is a gift—accept it. Did your teenage son attend a new program for vocational training, and transition beautifully to the new facility within the first week? It is a gift—accept it. Did your child enter your life, unannounced, unexpected, and bring a host of special blessings into your home? He is a gift—accept him.

Imagine the gifts that autism has bestowed upon those who are personally living with it. While many of us spent our teenage years focused on the opposite sex, fashion, and friends, our autistic peers were often already busy creating some of the most fascinating contributions to our modern world. Free from the social mandates that command us to fit in, to be cool, to look right, to crave attention, and to belong, autistic teens are sometimes better equipped to focus intensively on their passion, their life's purpose, their greatest inspiration. Of course, some regret that they could not adequately navigate the social rigors of teenage-dom. But many others simply pity those of us who focused so heavily on fitting in and making friends instead of making a difference.

It is often speculated that Albert Einstein himself was somewhere on the high end of the autism spectrum, possibly having Asperger's Syndrome. We will never know for certain if he was, in fact, autistic, but it is fair to say that had he been born today, he would most likely have been diagnosed during his preschool years. Albert Einstein had such poor organizational skills and was a lousy student—he failed math! He displayed a host of bizarre social behaviors and personal preferences. Yet from his mind sprang some of the most pivotal concepts in human history. All this is not to overshadow his compassionate philosophies on love, learning, human relationships, and so much more. Was Albert Einstein in need of a cure? I rather doubt it. Certainly, not all autistic children will grow up to be Einsteins, and surely, it is reasonable to seek a cure. But by acknowledging the possibility that lying dormant deep within your own child, a living fragment of the very same condition that fertilized Albert Einstein's genius is there, you can perhaps view your child's autism as a gift. Accept the gift of autism in your child's life. It will shift your perspective on your child's life and the possibilities within it.

AFFIRMATION: ACCEPTING THE GIFT

It is certainly hard to find the "gift" in autism sometimes. Even thinking about it as a gift can challenge me deeply. Yet inside, I know that my child with autism is a gift.

I know that many, many generations of people before me have unwittingly been hosts to people with autism. Of those with autism, many have left remarkable gifts behind them that continue to enhance the beauty and splendor of our world.

For the beautiful art that exists because of those special artists, I thank someone with autism. For the beautiful music created by those gifted musicians, I thank someone with autism. For the advances in medicine, science, and technology that I utilize daily, created by those focused on societal change, I thank someone with autism.

For whenever a gift is given, the right way to respond is not to balk in the face of generosity or complain that the gift is not what I asked for, but to simply say thank you.

Today, my heart accepts the gifts that people with autism bring into my life.

Today, to each of them, I say thank you.

Today, to my own child, I say thank you.

CHAPTER FOUR

MAKING PEACE WITH AUTISM

❤ How you can live within the contradiction: working to lessen the obstacles of autism while simultaneously accepting the autistic individual

❤ Affirmation: Making Peace With Autism

"Peace is a daily, a weekly, a monthly process, gradually changing opinions, slowly eroding old barriers, quietly building new structures."
-John F. Kennedy

"Having the wisdom to face the truth will bring us closer to peace."
-Melody Beattie

Peace. Just hearing the word automatically conjures images of great sages and political activists, of wars and treaties and sanctuaries. We think of Gandhi. We think of Jimmy Carter. We think of the Middle East. But we do not think of autism. Indeed, for many of us, the prospect of peace in the Middle East seems more realistic than the concept of making peace with autism! "Forgive my child's captor? Never," we quip with raw, heartfelt emotion. And so our resistance to peace persists. We persist in our viewpoint that autism is the great enemy, one to be exorcised from our children's bodies, minds, and spirits until at last, a perfect, pristine, and sparkling healthy child is left. We employ, out of absolute caring, every reasonable method that offers a glimpse of hope. We cram loads of vitamins and supplements down them, enforce rigid methods of behavior intervention upon them, and subject them to hundreds of therapeutic exercises, all jointly orchestrated for a single worthy purpose—to eliminate the characteristics of autism. But it is not autism that needs our attention. Our children need our attention. We push to annihilate autism entirely, one child at a time, until it exists no more. Sometimes this drive to destroy autism is fueled by unprecedented love for the child who has it. Often, the drive to destroy autism masquerades as love, but is really the harsh, unfiltered product of emotional pain that the disorder brought into our lives when we learned it was here with us to stay. We don't want it to stay. And so we fight it with all our being, and peace eludes us.

Of the many lessons you might learn from this book, making peace with autism is absolutely the most important. It's the most fundamental to progress, and the greatest catalyst for success for your child. And it's the one that nobody else dares to talk about, because it isn't an intervention you can bottle, structure, or sell, and it isn't something that everyone wants to hear—nor is the truth behind this message necessarily a popular one. But it's absolutely critical to your child's well-being, and if I'm to do my job well as an ethical, autism expert in this world, I need to tell you about it. So listen closely. In my years of working as an autism professional, meeting child after child, family after family, *I have never found a true success story where there is tremendous or ongoing unrest, rejection, or resistance to the presence of autism.* I'll repeat this for emphasis: I have never found a true success story where there is tremendous or ongoing unrest, rejection, or resistance to the presence of autism. People who are at war within themselves over how to react to their child's autism, and people who are filled with confusion over their child's autism in the long term deny themselves and their children health, balance, and joy. They focus too hard on the sidelines, and not enough on the main event. Most alarmingly, they inadvertently deny their own children—the very ones they love the most—the opportunity to become winners in the autism race. Today, if you have carried with you any discord, unrest, or painful confusion about your child's life with autism (and surely, we all have), you may take this chapter as an invitation to release it.

What would it mean in your life if the very thought of autism brought a tremendous sense of acceptance, peace, and serenity to you? What if, instead of conjuring sad, angry, conflicted, or sorrowful emotions, it brought forth joyous memories of your child breaking personal barriers, connecting with you in love, and moving past the obstacles that were once laid at his feet? You can make that change, and although it might take more than a moment, it can begin right here, right now.

Making peace with autism is not about ridding your child of disabilities and differences; it is about honoring your child's abilities and unique spirit.

Making peace with autism is not a passive, lazy, or timid act. It's not for sissies, the weak, or the faint at heart. It means working harder than anyone else to provide your child the most aggressive, intensive, comprehensive, and effective intervention imaginable *not because you seek to expel your child's autism, but because you seek to illuminate her spirit.* While your actions may be the same as another parent's to a child with autism, what will set you apart is your ability to see past the autism, past the obstacles, and recognize both the obvious and hidden treasures buried deep within your bright, beautiful child. When you can do this, day after day, week after week, month after month, and finally year after year, then you will have made peace with autism. When you have made peace with autism, it will be as if the weight of the world (which you are probably feeling on your neck and back at this very moment) has been not just lifted from you, but *dissolved* entirely. You will notice that things in your child's life—and yours—seem to fall into place with ease. Achievements will bloom, and struggles lessen. You will see a shift in your child's entire way of being in this world, and it can happen overnight if you are open to allowing it! People and resources enter the picture that were not there for you before. Remarkably, you'll begin to perceive a change in how you are viewed, treated, and responded to by teachers, therapists, and other parents of special needs children. You will rise above your prior view of autism, and you will find that soon, other parents are coming to you, calling you, seeking advice from you, whom they perceive as "having it together" more than they do. But the secret is, you have nothing that they do not already have, except for having made peace with autism. That single difference in perception, understanding, and acceptance is a critical part of what it takes to make your child's potential flourish and grow into tangible success. It is to stop obsessing about the autism. It is perhaps even to stop thinking regularly about the autism. It is to start loving your child as a *whole* child, and *get on with the work.*

Are you someone who, like so many of us, gets bogged down by the negative side of it all? That's okay—you're human! The goal is not to forget or ignore that your child has autism. We must on certain levels focus on autism in order to create the ideal instructional and environmental learning conditions for children with autism. But we must not do this when we are looking at our children. Stop the mental dialogue that derails you from being a parent, and insists that you become a data-hoarding, obsessive, autism junkie. Yes, I did say "junkie." There are parents out there who become so consumed by their child's autism, that chasing new treatments and possible causes can become like a drug. While this is fairly typical at the beginning of the autism journey, it is not generally healthy or effective as a long-term approach. Somewhere along the way, obsessive searching becomes non-productive, even counterproductive. Instead of chasing external information, focus your energies on the very core of who your child is. What abilities, goals, and successes would you like to see shining out from within her today? How can you and the professionals in her life bring out those qualities? Can they, in fact, be brought out from within her? If not, what can be? Do absolutely everything within your power to *address* your child's autism. But stop trying to find something to *blame* for your child's autism. Blame is the product of anger, and anger, when carried long term and/or buried, is the catalyst for discord, chaos, and eventually, illness. If you are ill, you are not at your best to help your child. And since you are the most powerful resource your child has, you must protect yourself in order to protect your child. Do not let the anger and blame consume you, for it will eventually consume you if you continue to dance in the flames of its fire! The current witch-hunt for something to blame for autism is effectively brewing two very dangerous things in our autism community:

1. It is systematically distracting loving, caring parents and professionals from effectively and aggressively acting with comprehensive intervention from all angles for their child right now,

2. It is depriving children of precious, irreplaceable intervention time that is never to be made up for in the future.

When you are at peace with autism, the source of your child's autism still matters to you—but it takes the backseat to swift, aggressive action. When you are at peace with autism, instead of searching day in and day out for what to blame, you are busy *serving* your child with what *works*. Initially, these two schools of seem mutually exclusive, and although it is possible, it is not common to find a parent who is focusing heavily on the blame aspect of autism *and* simultaneously focusing on the intervention aspect. This is because the motivations diverge—blame is based in fear, active intervention is based in love. That is the scary part. Most parents who are focusing heavily on tracing the source of their child's autism do not *realize* that their energy is being diminished in the area of intervention. Far from a criticism, this observation has been made time and time and time again by those of us working in the professional arena. We see parents *watching* autism, mesmerized all its possible causes, or fixated on one potential cause, not actively treating autism with a whole-child approach, which includes more than experimental treatments to rid the body of the autism source. We seek to draw parents away from watching the car wreck on the side of the road, and urge them gently to watch where they are driving their children along the autism intervention road.

Perhaps a cure for autism will be found. Perhaps it will not. Regardless, in your child's lifetime, every single moment and iota of energy that you can spare on his behalf will be effectively, wisely, and responsibly used when it is focused on active education, skill building, and intervention. Because in the end, if a cure hasn't been found by the time your child is an adult, then whatever skills he has developed will be all he has to help him navigate this world. And to build those skills, you must work hard, now. Do not let fear take you to a place of distraction—there is no time for that. Instead, let it take you to a place of love, of hard work, and of effective strategizing for your child. What caused your child's autism? It is with heartache and compassion that I humbly tell you, I do not know. But whatever caused it, it is in the past. What can you do to change the course of your child's life experience with autism? That is joyfully known—you can provide him the most effective, powerful intervention possible! What you can do for your child with autism is in the present! You cannot change the past. You have carte blanche to change the present! And perhaps most powerfully, when you act in the present, the changes you make will influence your child's short- and long-term future. Take control of the present, and let go of the past. The scientists will handle the search for the cure. The researchers will handle the search for a cause. And parents—*your job is to search for your own child's greatest strengths*. Find the right teachers, find the right schools, find the right therapists and support staff and consultants—find the right fit for your child. Do this now. You will do him more good this way than with all other efforts combined.

Go ahead. Now you get it. You must make peace with autism.

AFFIRMATION:
MAKING PEACE WITH AUTISM

This is a turning point for me. I have learned that my efforts can serve my child best when they are focused on the present, not the past. I know that this is true, and I embrace this truth today!

I can apply the concept of peace right here, right now, and make peace with autism. In my heart, today I choose to release the unrest, the unsettled confusion, anger, resentment, and worry that comes with my old perspective on autism. I release these emotions, and in doing so, I create space for peace to occupy my heart. This peace gives me feelings of love and serenity, and a view of tranquil roads ahead even through the bumpy parts of life. This peace belongs not just to me, but to my child, who needs me desperately right now to work on his behalf. By making the choice to lift my head from the fog of blame, I am making the choice to lift my child to a place of better success. My child is worth it, and so I affirm that I choose to make peace with autism.

In creating a sense of peace with autism, there are good things I can count on:

-I can count on appreciating the beauty and worth within my child

-I can count on myself to move ahead in the right direction for my child

-I can count on others around me to respond to my needs and the needs of my child better than ever before

-I can count on my child's future being as strong and bright as the peace I choose to create within myself

Today, for the first time, the second time, or the hundredth time, I affirm with great joy and determination that I am at peace with autism!

CHAPTER FIVE

YOUR CHANCE TO SHINE

❤ The key secrets to being the most powerful, effective, and positive presence in the life of someone with autism

❤ Affirmation: Embracing My Role

"You have powers you never dreamed of. You can do things you never thought you could do. There are no limitations in what you can do except the limitations of your own mind."
-Darwin P. Kingsley

If making peace with autism is the spiritual backbone of parenting a child with autism, then being equipped with the know-how and strategies to bring that peace into tangible action for your child's best interest is the physical backbone. This chapter is the "meat and potatoes" part of the book. Here, you will learn exactly how to act as the most powerful, effective, and positive presence in the life of someone with autism. I hope that this chapter does something for you that no other autism resource has. Instead of telling you *what* to do, my goal is to teach you *how to decide for yourself what to do, when to do it, and why you should do it.* Whether you are a parent, teacher, sibling, or friend, you can take these tools and apply them daily to make a difference in the life of someone with autism. While there are many other practical ways to help address autism needs, these twenty categories encompass the key concepts that make other outside practical steps obvious, understood, and easy to apply. The most effective tools in autism intervention, whether mentioned specifically here or not, can all be traced back, on some level, to one of these twenty keys. Using this information can help you to *think critically, decide effectively,* and *act with confidence* on behalf of your student or child. Some of these keys are specific in nature, while others are general concepts and belief systems. Combined, they make for a very powerful approach to intervention. And, since we've got a lot to cover, I'm going to jump right into it.

The 20 Key Secrets To Positive Autism Intervention

1) **Know Your Child Inside and Out.** Who else will? It's wonderful to have teachers who are really on top of your child's needs and behaviors, but if you don't know exactly what your child's strengths, weaknesses, preferences, and dislikes are, then she's not getting complete assistance from you. Figure out what makes your child tick, tock, and tucker out. If you pick your child up from speech therapy to learn that she had a meltdown over the expectation to make the "ah" sound, find out why, even if the therapist doesn't know. Ask questions and probe for details. A-ha! You might discover that the computer program used to encourage her has a high-pitched "ding" noise that sounds when the child gets something correct—and your daughter hates those types of sounds. You might find that a Barney doll was on the shelf of the therapy room, and deduce that she was probably distracted because she wanted to play with her favorite character. Learn to be the "Sherlock Holmes" of your child's inner workings, and you'll do a great service to her every time. Realize that sometimes, a child is just a child, and she may be cranky, tired, or just having a tough time mastering some of the obstacles that come with her autism. But don't give up. Consider the possibilities before chalking something up to autism itself or to being "nothing."

2) **Claim Your Power.** Stop giving away your power to the other people in your child's life! It does not matter if your child's program is developed by someone with eight Ph.D.'s or is the most reputable, sought-after program in town. You still have the power to stay involved and make choices that benefit your child!

Claiming your power does not mean you must become an expert on all things autism. It *does* mean that you must know how to effectively work *with* the experts. Working with talented, knowledgeable, experienced professionals is a great gift to you and your child. But too often, I see parents taken aback by big-name professionals or programs, and they simply stop making choices and hand over control to the professional. Often, it's a combination of factors that lead to this type of role shift. The professional is generally sincerely caring and qualified, and trust is placed in that professional for good reasons. The professional speaks confidently, based on repeated experience, and the parents, who are going through this for the first time, feel that the professional knows best. This is very often true! Sometimes, parents are simply overwhelmed and exhausted, and lack the energy to do anything more than what's asked of them. In other cases, professionals are very assertive and persuasive, hoping to facilitate the best services for a child, but come across as an authority figure over the parents. A professional should certainly be an authority in his field of expertise—but not an authority over the parents! Either way, the parent/professional roles can sometimes go awry when parents blindly accept (without understanding, agreeing with, or simply questioning out of interest or uncertainty) the decisions being made about their own child's life.

The best professionals understand the *balance* that is required between parents, professionals, and final decisions. And so do the best parents. Great professionals care nothing for the game of intimidation, control, and power plays. True professionalism and quality in the world of autism goes way beyond knowledge, experience, and background. In addition to those highly valuable assets, you want to work with professionals who value your thoughts, questions, and concerns, and who address each of those things with the understanding that this is your first time going through this. If you already knew exactly what to do, how to do it, and had time to do it, then you wouldn't have a need for professionals! Rather than handing off your child's intervention to others, select professionals who involve you, listen to you, and ask you to participate through incorporating additional interventions outside the office. Make sure your professionals communicate with you openly and regularly, do not dismiss your concerns as silly or ignorant, and display a genuine interest in your child. Most importantly, choose professionals who possess these qualities *and* are effective for your child's needs within a reasonable amount of time. By the same token, professionals are like to work with parents who are proactive, educated about their child's disability, thoughtful and respectful communicators, appreciative, cooperative, and have realistic, reasonable expectations. Nothing is worse for a professional than working hard all day long to genuinely make a difference in a child's life and knowing that the parents will take that child home and do little for him. The "that's what I pay you for" and "fix my child for me" mentalities are not only offensive to professionals, but they are also counter-productive to your own child's progress. Claim your power, use your power, and apply it to change your child's life for the better!

3) **Identify Strong, Meaningful Motivators.** I can no longer count how many times I've been invited to observe a child in his classroom to help resolve an

academic, social, or behavioral problem, only to find
that there is no problem—with what the *student* is
doing! Parents and teachers, listen up. If you typically
have a reward system that consists of handing out an
M&M, token, or star for a chart, and you find that an
autistic student is not responding as you'd like him to,
change your motivators!! If your son loves lining
Hot wheels cars up in large numbers and teachers are
stuck trying to extinguish a bothersome, disruptive
behavior that involves loudly blurting out answers
without raising his hand, bring in what works! Send a
collection of the cars to be kept at school, and set an
expectation with the teachers that is appropriate for
your child. For example, based on his specific abilities
to exercise self-control, personal restraint, and to comply
with verbal directions to raise his hand, you might allow
him to keep a special chart on his desk. Each time that
he raises his hand, waits his turn, and offers a reasonable
(not necessarily correct, depending on your goal)
answer, he may mark off his earning one more car (or
two, or three, depending upon how many chances he
has to be called on fairly throughout the day). You want
the reward to be not just conceptually meaningful, but
practically meaningful as well. If he loves lining up
masses of cars, you aren't doing him any favors by giving
him four or five at the end of the day, so make your
reward work accordingly. Throughout the day, he can
earn the right to access cars. At the end of the day, he
may line them up and play with them for five minutes.
If your child is a sucker for the Wendy's fast food logo,
then print out paper logos and reward the child with
that. If he loves Australian sand sharks, buy him some
little plastic ones from an aquarium gift shop or website,

and reward him with those. If your child demonstrates no clear connection to specific motivators, get creative. Does he drag a silk houseplant around at home? Bring it to school! Does she laugh with glee at the neighbor's dog? Arrange a meet-up! Does he linger in the lunch-room, gazing at the beautifully linear stacks of lunch trays on their cart? Let him help stack! There is no law that says your child has to have the same mundane rewards as every other kid in the class, and there are an infinite number of motivators for each child, if only you will use your imagination. Encourage your child's teachers to incorporate his personal interests into the classroom reward system, and absolutely do the same at home! Get creative, and get your child motivated. It's that simple.

4) **Learn To Do Voice Impersonations.** You don't really have to impersonate anyone, but you do need to get good at modifying the tone of your voice in extremely varying ways. Why, you ask? Because autism impacts communication significantly, and your child may or may not catch that whole phrase you just threw out at him— but he *will* more likely understand, based on the tone of your voice, what *kind* of interaction you are presenting him with. This is also a great way to instill social skills. You're helping him to read emotions based on other, more consistent factors than cause and effect (also very important to teach). Is he up for a treat, or in for a scolding? Is his choice to turn the TV on during dinner okay, or not okay? Was his perfect handwriting page that came home from school today impressive to you, or just the same as a note about field trip money? Let him know, in part, through the tone of your voice. Not only can this help strengthen his receptive communication

skills, but it can also help motivate him to elicit the positive, not negative, tone based on his behavior choices. Your voice can be a reward in and of itself, when used properly, as a form of praise! Dramatically changing your tone of voice can be extremely valuable and critical when it comes to controlling unsafe or violent behaviors. My typically sweet, sing-song voice quickly drops to the "Mr. T" range—and is as loud as he would be in person—when I see that a child is engaging in something dangerous. You might think I'm being funny or exaggerating, but I'm not! It's a skill my mentors Marian Joiner and Valerie Trinklein taught me. In extreme cases where biting, clawing, hitting, throwing heavy objects, or other unsafe behaviors occur , I really change my demeanor, voice, and overall presence. In a lineup, after hearing my "safety" voice, you'd think a burly male bodybuilder was the source of that sound—not me! And that is precisely the point. Sometimes, this shocking, unexpected voice is all you need to prevent something negative from happening and avoid the need for physical restraint entirely. In these extreme cases, once your safety voice has successfully interrupted the potentially unsafe act, you must follow through and immediately redirect the stressed student to something better, more appropriate, and easier for him to negotiate without stress. Tone of voice—and the facial expression that goes with it—is a valuable asset when you need to go a step beyond "standard" communication, at home or in the classroom. Instead of just letting your tone of voice "happen" based on how you feel, deliberately manipulate your voice and face to achieve a desired result.

5) **Take Stock of Your Child's Strengths and Weaknesses.** What are your child's greatest strengths? You should be capitalizing upon them! What are his greatest weaknesses? You should be working to strengthen them! You don't diminish weakness by ignoring it, or worrying about it, but by actively building skills that inspire strengths. By drawing out the strengths that already exist and activating them, the whole world suddenly becomes brighter, easier, and more navigable for your child. Too often, we focus on what our children with autism do not do. We look at what they *do not* have so intensely that we forget about all the great qualities, skills, and capabilities that they do have. We say, "She doesn't speak. She doesn't tie her shoes yet. She doesn't hold her own fork yet. She doesn't play with other kids yet." Well, what *does* she do? How can you be a powerful force for positive change for your child? Focus on enhancing the qualities that shine in your child just as much as you emphasize diminishing the behaviors that aren't ideal.

Throughout my schooling, I struggled a lot with math. I didn't get it, didn't want to get it—I hated it, in fact! If my school day had consisted of intense "math intervention" all day long, focusing solely on combating my weakness, I think I would have probably curled up into a ball under my desk and cried! Instead, I had a diverse academic day that was filled with various activities and opportunities. Math was an important part of my education, so it was not ignored. But math was not the *only* aspect of my education. I excelled in English, French, debate, history, and anything else that didn't involve numbers and equations. I was placed in higher level English classes, added to the newspaper staff, praised for my advanced writing and speaking abilities, and for math, I remained in basic courses that matched my needs. Now think about your child—how diverse and balanced is his intervention right now? Is every ounce of effort focused on his weaknesses, and is that draining and aggravating him daily? *Find a balance.* Let your child *enjoy* aspects of his intervention. Some aspects of intervention are bound to be unpleasant to your child, and that's okay; that may even be a good thing, because it teaches him adaptability, flexibility, and cooperation. Making it through non-preferred activities teaches our children with autism to realize, "Hey, I'm no fan of this activity, but I know that when I get it done right, I can move on to something else." Our children learn to survive the ups and downs that come with life, and that's more important to children with autism than to any other group of children! We do not want to raise our children with autism to be spoiled, thinking that the world revolves around their desires, training them falsely to believe that when things don't go their way, a meltdown is in order to get things back on track. But don't expect *more* tolerance for a stressful education from your autistic child than you would from yourself!

By emphasizing my strengths, my education groomed me beautifully for my career, which includes frequent public speaking, effective communication with parents, professionals, and organizations, and of course, being an author! If your child absolutely loves dinosaurs and possesses a wealth of knowledge about them, don't dismiss this as a "perseveration" or "splinter skill." When typical people like you and I have a passion for a specific subject area, these things are called "hobbies," "interests," or "passions." Are autistic people not allowed the same? An interest *becomes* perseverative when it interferes with someone's ability to effectively focus and act on other appropriate things. That does not make the area of interest itself inappropriate; it makes the behavior of *not adapting properly to the situation* inappropriate. Act to diminish and replace the behavior, then, and not the interest! Your child's interest in dinosaurs, antique cars, Japanese animation, carnivorous plants, or PVC pipes (all real-life examples) is a *strength*. Use it to your child's advantage. Work it into lessons, rewards, opportunities, and help him succeed through what he loves.

6) **Don't Teach What He Can't See.** Stop relying on words and verbal cues alone to work for your child with autism. Include them, use them, but by all means, support them with visual aides. Use calendars—simple, picture-filled calendars—that help children understand the events in their lives. If your child does not fully comprehend verbal directions and communication , you can convey complete messages to him by using visual cues! There are plenty of great resources out there to help you learn how to design effective picture schedules and calendars. But in addition to knowing *how* to use these things, I want you yo understand *why* it's beneficial to use these things. Sure, we all know that visual cues help children with autism because processing differences can make verbal directions a sticky issue for some. But why is this the case, and what is it about the picture or schedule that helps? If you understand the qualities in the process that make it worthwhile, you're much more likely to implement other creative visual prompts that you come up with on your own!

Sometimes, a person with autism has difficulty processing not only the transition that's currently on the table, but also struggles with how the next step fits in with everything else going on in his or her life. Often, parents and teachers don't understand the underlying issue that makes visual transitioning so effective, and as a result, they don't plan comprehensive daily or weekly schedules that truly meet the child's specific transitioning or processing needs. Is the idea of spelling out the student's schedule a week in advance too overwhelming and organized for teachers and/or parents? Then that may be part of the problem! The term "visual support" almost implies that it's there just to help, but isn't a major factor. Don't assume the visual cues or supports are just the icing on the cake. Instead, view them as critical. A student who struggles with transitions sometimes *requires* the concrete, identifiable outline of what's coming next in order to help manage anxieties over transitioning. If he has no idea what's happening and when, then it's not surprising that he's stressed and resistant to getting up in the morning, going to school, moving from homeroom activities to music or P.E., etc. While some of the struggles may have to do with the content of the activities themselves and will need to be addressed separately, simply giving your child the power to know what's happening in his daily life can yield a significant improvement.

Imagine being asked to go to "work" daily, but not being given any further information: which days you go, for how long, where you will be working, or what the expectations will be for you to do that day! You might anxiously wonder: Will I ever get to go home? When? How soon will this part of my day be over? Is there something I am expected to do next? What will that be? Will I like it? Can I do it? Will it finish? Will I see my husband tonight? *Telling* the student with autism may not be enough. Visually *showing* the student can be a lifeline to calm and comfort. He will be set up for success by understanding what's happening, when, and what to expect afterwards. Do this every day, all day, and tensions over transitioning can be minimized greatly. Take pictures of everything; from your home's front door, to the backseat where your child sits in the car, to your child's speech therapist. Whenever possible, I strongly recommend actual, personal photos over-generalized computer program icons and materials. These cartoons, sketches, and mass-produced photos may work in some cases, but are not *as* valuable to your child as realistic representations of items and people that she/he comes in contact with daily and already has some experience with. Use these photos in combination with brief, clear verbal and written support. I'll give you an example. Let's say your child has difficulty organizing and preparing for school in the morning (and who are we kidding—some of us *without* autism have trouble getting things together in the rush before work). You might create a simple, clear schedule to help him understand both *what* is expected and *when* it is expected. The morning schedule could look something like this, written on large, easy to read card stock:

1) [Photo of your child brushing teeth] Brush teeth

2) [Photo of your child dressing] Get dressed

3) [Photo of your child brushing hair] Brush hair

4) [Photo of food at your kitchen table] Eat breakfast

5) [Photo of your child's lunch bag] Get my lunch

6) [Photo of your child's backpack] Get my backpack

7) [Photo of seat in car] Get in car, or buckle up to ride!

Of course, you will naturally have steps that may differ from these, and in a different order as well. If you prefer, you may choose to offer photos of the objects themselves (e.g., the toothbrush at the sink, the clothing on the bed) rather than action shots. It's truly up to you. If your child has been forgetting his lunch bag, or neglecting to brush his hair, helping him clearly identify when it's time to take care of this responsibility in comparison to other morning duties can help him remember. The concept of "first _____, then _____" can really help make sense of things, as well as the concept of "next, _____." Now that you have designed your picture schedule, find a noticeable, centrally-located area to keep it for your child's easy access. This could be on your refrigerator, posted on the wall just outside your child's bedroom door, or on the bathroom mirror, for example, depending upon what works for your child. When morning comes and it's time to get up, you'll help your child find his way to the schedule (soon, he'll understand it as part of his routine, and go on his own) and begin. If your child reads, then have him tell you what's happening. If not, you read out loud and allow your child to fill in the blanks when you point to the picture specifying the activity. So if your child reads, he would tell you, "Number one: brush teeth," and then get started brushing his teeth. If your child does not read and can articulate a word, you'll say to him, "Number one: brush _____," and point to the picture. Your child will respond, "teeth!" Note that for this type of work, you may choose a different type of photo as well, so that your child has a clear sense of what to say. In other words, if you want your child to say "teeth," it may be too much to ask for him to assume "teeth" from a photo of the toothbrush, and may be better served with an actual photo of teeth. If your child is nonverbal, you simply make sure he's watching as you guide him through the steps. Once teeth are brushed, you return to the schedule, say, "Number one is FINISHED," and treat number two the same way.

Once at school, a chart should outline the student's entire daily schedule in exactly the same fashion. This should be placed in a central location to the child as well—either on the side of the board or taped to the child's desk. Once #1 is finished, the child will check it off. This gives critical support to your student, who is now empowered by understanding what will happen at school, when it happens and in what order, and perhaps most importantly to this child, that school *ends* when the chart is completed each day! Additional picture

charts at home can outline therapies, meal times, homework expectations, the amount of TV your child can watch and in what order in relation to other at-home tasks. Now that you understand the nature of picture schedules, you can apply this technique virtually anywhere! Sometimes, actual photos are not necessary, but the visual support of having a schedule written down can still help. I advise parents to keep a mini dry-erase board with them everywhere (especially in the car), and to simply write out "spontaneous" schedules as needed to ease transitioning for things you may not have planned or anticipated. This dry-erase schedule can be created on a moment's notice, and can even help handle sticky situations that aren't a part of the normal routine. Here is an example: you don't have any after-school childcare and you need to bring your anxious child with you during an oil change for your car! You can whip up a quick schedule that reads, 1) Oil change for car [if your child does not know what an oil change is, that's okay—you can use the correct terminology and teach him to know where you're   going, or you can simplify the concept to something easier to grasp, like "Fix the car"]. 2) Read a book [Always keep a copy of your child's favorite book on hand in the car. It can serve as a familiar transition object *and* keep him occupied and happy for a few extra minutes when you're in a bind]. 3) Sit quietly. 4) Get a prize! [Make the prize something your child loves—be more specific than "prize" if need be, such as "get a dinosaur" or "get a new coloring book," or whatever works. Then follow through with the reward! 5) Go home!
Happy transitioning, everyone!

7) **Stop Slamming Your Child With "No."** How strong is your child's ability to adapt to transitions, new directions and assignments, and to put down something of interest? If it's not great, then I hope I have your attention here. Trouble in these areas of development is par for the course with a diagnosis of autism. But the degree and extent to which your child struggles to handle these things can be a direct reflection of the approach taken to help him. For kids with autism, saying "no" all the time just doesn't work. It might seem to work at first, but just wait until your child gets older, and the problems may start to surface. Why is this true? Giving children with autism a sense of what is not okay to do will never teach them what they *can* do instead. It happens every day, thousands of times in homes and classrooms across America and beyond. A child with autism is flapping his hands with glee, watching the movement up and down, up and down, and the teacher says, "Stop flapping!" The child halts briefly. The teacher is satisfied. Five minutes later, the child is flapping again, and the teacher's level of tolerance is shrinking. "I told you, stop flapping! Why don't you listen? Stop flapping!" At home, the child sits down at the dinner table to eat with family. Just after taking a bite, he loves the flavor and flaps his hands. Mom and dad have been trying to get him to stop flapping during dinner for weeks now, and mom says, "Cut it out! We do not do that at the dinner table!" The child looks at mom, looks at the expression on dad's face (we all remember that daunting expression, don't we?), and stops. Until he starts again.

Sure, the child's hand flapping is attributed to autism. But his noncompliance with your request to stop it *may not* be a result of autism alone. It may be the result of incomplete guidance and teaching on the part of the adult. Instead of being told no, what this child needs is a *replacement behavior*, and preferably one that can qualify as an *incompatible behavior* as well. A replacement behavior is exactly what it sounds like: a desirable behavior designed to replace a less desirable behavior. If your child is busy riding his bike, for example, then he is no longer kicking the new azalea bush you just planted so that he can watch the loose blooms fall off. The behavior of kicking the azalea bush has been replaced with bike riding. An incompatible behavior is one that, when used as a replacement behavior, makes it impossible for your child to simultaneously continue with the original, undesired behavior. This is what our friend the hand flapper needs right now. Instead of being told "don't flap at dinner," he needs specific, detailed instruction on what behavior is expected. To get a child to stop hitting the walls of the hallway as you travel from music class back to your academic classroom, you might purposely bring along some books of yours and choose to have him hold your things down the hallway. The stack of a few books should be just cumbersome enough (not unreasonably heavy) that he'll need to use both hands to carry them. When he's following through on what he *should* be doing, he cannot be simultaneously hitting the walls! In that example, nobody used the word "no," drew attention to the wrong behavior, or upset the child. In a respectful, fast, and effective way, the undesirable behavior was stopped, and instead, you've now created a special opportunity for this child to feel good about helping and *receive praise for doing the right thing!*

Now back to our hand-flapping friend. You can tell this child, for example, "pick up your fork." When he picks up his fork, you can instruct him, "take a bite!" As he complies, you praise and clearly confirm what the expectation is: "Good eating! It's time to eat!" If he picks up the fork and flaps with the fork in his hand, preventing him from putting food on his fork, then you need to use an incompatible behavior, like, "Hands touch the table," then, "Next, food on fork—go quickly!" At school, instead of "no flapping," the teacher can say, "Pick up your pencil," then, "Write your name." If she runs into flapping with the pencil in hand, she may choose to modify her direction, or offer a different option entirely, like "Hands in pockets, please." If his hands are in his pockets, then they cannot be flapping next to his ears! Please be careful to direct children only with expectations that are reasonable and doable—do not set a student up for failure by telling him to keep his hands in his pockets, only to find that he *has* no pockets on his pants that day. I once made this mistake accidentally, and felt terrible at the glimpse of my sweet, endearing, compliant student, bewildered by my elusive request as he solved the problem of no pockets by sliding his hands tightly down the sides of his pants! Some common autistic behaviors can effectively be managed during classroom time through collaborative parent/teacher planning. Teachers, ask that your student's mom always dress him in pants with pockets for school. Parents, ask that teachers remember to have a plan of action that will comprehensively and effectively interrupt the behaviors you seek to extinguish. And be reasonable and patient! If you know that your child flaps his hands during every free moment, then don't

expect the teacher to magically transform school into a
"Flap-Free Zone!" By the same token, teachers, if
something is working well for you at school, be sure to
communicate your successful strategy so that parents
can provide consistency at home. Don't wait for an IEP
meeting to say, "we stopped Joey's flapping during
reading circle entirely by asking him to help hold the
book while the teacher reads!" Let parents know that
what works for this student is putting something else in
his hands. They'll thank and love you for the insider
tips! Apply these replacement behavior strategies to
everything. For transitions, don't just tell your student
it's time to stop one activity, or name the thing that
comes next. Provide an object of transition and give him
a direction on where to put it, like, "Art is next! Take
this paintbrush to Mrs. Stellano!" If holding the object
is either not possible (rare—you can always find
something to transition with), or more than what's
necessary for this student's level of ability, show the
child a picture of something fun and exciting in the next
room: "Music is next. Look—it's a big drum! It's your
turn for the big drum!" Again, make sure you set the
child up for success. Don't promise a turn first on the
big drum if you haven't coordinated this with the other
teacher! Nothing is worse than *negating* the transition
process by making empty promises that work on *your*
end of the deal, but leave the child and other staff
member struggling to manage! Getting the student out
of your room, home, or car at all costs is not the goal.
It's getting him to smoothly and effectively move on to
the next expectation that matters. Learn to use
replacement behaviors and transition objects instead of
simply saying "no." You can then reserve "no" for big,

important safety issues when "no" really means "no," and you don't have time to expect the child to process something else. Your life will probably be a lot easier— and so will your child's!

8) **Eliminate Errors.** Research shows that a child with autism who accidentally learns the wrong answer to something may take *up to ten repetitions or more of the correct answer* to undo the inaccurate learning. This is attributed to processing differences, and means that your child might retain the wrong information for the right reasons! What would be the "right" reason to retain a wrong answer? Learning error-filled lessons, of course! From ABA therapy we have extracted a powerful concept in autism teaching—the concept of errorless learning. Essentially, this approach is simple. It means that when teaching your child or student a new skill, the learning environment and expectations are deliberately set up for the child's success on the first try! With error-less learning, we choose to keep the learning process simplified, minimal, and highly structured. Think of it as taking a "Zen" approach to teaching! This can be executed by, say, giving your child only one option to choose from—the *correct* option—when asking him to "point to yellow." Use a clear work surface, preferably a small, non-cluttered school desk, but any appropriate area will work. For this particular example, your child will first need to understand and be able to execute the direction to "point." Rather than offering a line up of all the colors, you present your child only with yellow, and construct the scenario such that he can only *choose* yellow. When he gets it correct, you will praise him joyfully—and repeat! Several repetitions later, the child has successfully—and painlessly—mastered the goal of

recognizing the color yellow. Next, you will move on to teaching the color green. Now, you will provide two choices, yellow (now known and recognized by the child) and green (unknown; the subject of the lesson). Withhold the yellow card by keeping it further away from your child than the green card, which should be right up front and center within reach. Given the direction, "Point to GREEN," your child may make a lunge for yellow out of habit and due to communication deficits—so watch out! If this happens, remember that the #1 goal here is to set the child up for success on the first try. Yank that yellow card off the desk before she/he has a chance to get it incorrect, and redirect so that your child does point to the green card. Praise, and repeat! If she/he gets it right the first time naturally, even better, but you've got to have catlike reflexes in order to make this work, just in case. You can introduce colors, letters, numbers, words, animals, facial expression cards— almost anything in this fashion one by one until all are mastered. Then, you'll need to make sure your student can generalize what she/he's learned in the controlled setting. Pointing to a yellow card is a great way to teach the concept of yellow, but do follow through and make sure your child can identify yellow in a real-life context as well! Don't assume that just because she/he did it for you at the desk when prompted, she/he will do it again for someone else, outside, pointing to a taxi cab! I recently viewed a news program that presented a segment about autism. They were filming a major autism treatment center that's known nationwide, and I watched the clip as the teacher/therapist had about six different color cards spread across the child's desk. She said, "Point to green," and the boy went straight for red. She did nothing to intercept the inaccurate choice, and repeated, "Point to GREEN," with stronger emphasis on "green." Again, the boy pointed to red. The rest of the viewing audience was probably thinking, "Oh, he's so cute, and isn't that wonderful—he's learning his colors and the teacher is so nice," and I was thinking, "Uh-oh—that's not errorless!" Through no fault of his own, the boy had already linked the word "green" with the color "red," and she was going to have one heck of a time undoing that, and it could have been avoided to begin with. Be careful when utilizing errorless learning—or any other teaching tactic, for that matter—that you *incorporate the core concept* as needed. It's great to be creative and use bits and pieces of methods to help support a unique approach for your student, but if the core advantage of errorless learning is the "errorless" part, don't bother setting up unless you're ready to follow through!

9) **Use Your Intuition.** Intuition is not listed as one of the major autism intervention strategies today, but it should be. Is everyone telling you that a particular program is fantastic, but your gut just says, "I don't know why, but I just don't have a good feeling about this place?" Pay attention to that internal message, and follow it. What's worse than spending money, wasting time, and losing hope on a program that wasn't worth it in the end? Realizing that it could have been avoided if you'd just followed your intuition! Conversely, if nobody else is taking their child the playground three times a week to climb on the monkey bars, but you feel in your gut that you need to make time for this, go ahead! Your intuitive system is a powerful compass that can guide you to good decisions for your child. You might find, for

example, that on your third week of "monkey bar intervention," you meet a new mom whose typical son is your child's age and has the patience of Job when it comes to encouraging your child to participate in joint play or dialogue! Your intuition will never guide you to make a "bad" choice. It's true—"bad" decisions are made when we listen to the fear-based messages within us, not the genuinely intuitive messages. You gave birth to this child, you're raising this child—why would "mother knows best" *not* apply to you? Autism is a tricky path to navigate sometimes, and there are no set answers on how exactly to treat your child. Since there is no definite "right" or "wrong" on what path to take, then you need to feel comfortable doing what you believe is right for *your* child. Nobody can tell you this but you. What will happen to help you along? You will read, explore, and learn about strategies that other people have developed in the way of autism intervention. Some of these things will "click" with you, and you will pursue them. Others will feel unmatched to your situation, and you will dismiss them. It's that simple. Sometimes, like the monkey bar example, you will come up with things that guide you to help your child in a conventional or unconventional way. Your task is to hear your own recommendations for your own child and follow them.

10) **Use Your Brain.** Intuition is a powerful tool, but it usually works best in conjunction with your brain! Has anyone else noticed how many people are blindly following the trends in the autism world without exercising the critical thinking required to keep children safe and healthy? Of course, it takes two to tango, and unethical professionals are at the heart of some of the

worst autism scams yet uncovered. Have we come to a place of confusion so deep that we are willing to try anything, proposed by anyone, at any cost, to rid our children of autism? I certainly hope not. This is not to diminish the valiant efforts that caring parents are willing to make for their children. But in the interest of your child's future, learn how to separate the emotional feelings of *desperation* from the rational *guidance* of your mind as a responsible adult entrusted with making wise decisions for your child. Your choices affect his life positively or negatively, depending upon the course of action you choose. If you feel little hope or happiness at the thought of your child's autism, then I urge you to go back and read chapter four on making peace with autism. Read it and reread it again until you no longer feel as though your child's diagnosis is a dead end. And when you realize that your child is already "okay" exactly as she is, and that every improvement made by every intervention is a blessing that helps uncover her spirit and frees her, you will no longer feel the urge to throw away hundreds of thousands of dollars on sketchy—sometimes preposterous—claims from questionable programs to rid her of her autism. Simply put, use your brain. Does it sound too good to be true? It probably is. Is it heavily marketed with tear-jerking testimonials—but no solid data? Take note. Does it claim it can work for any child with autism? Watch out. Does it cost more than a car payment? Weigh the pro's and con's—and find out where that money goes. Can you or your child's teachers learn to implement it yourself? Find out why or why not, and if you have to pay a hefty fee for a short time to learn how to do it, research that, too. Do you absolutely need this professional or program in order to utilize this concept or style of intervention for your child? Decipher whether you are paying for a professional's personal expertise as designed individually for your child, or paying for a brand name that's mass marketed in a one-size-fits-all fashion. Testimonials and sharp looking web pages do not a sound intervention make! Be careful. *Caveat emptor* still applies, even in the world of autism. I'd say it applies *especially* to parents in the world of autism.

Parents, it's time to stop letting unsavory professionals, programs, and therapies rope you into acting as though you can't think for yourselves! Some may be unethical in luring you to their schemes, but most professionals are good, caring, and working sincerely to improve the quality of your child's life. Regarding those few bad seeds who have strayed from the unspoken guidelines of best practices, avoid them— and know that those of us who are really working hard for your kids want nothing to do with them, either! The only way to do this is by utilizing critical thinking. They're not going to tell you that they're not exactly all they claim to be. On the contrary, many doctors, therapists, and parents who start up these programs very sincerely *believe* in what they're doing. So be careful. Ask the right questions. Research it. Think about it. And if you need to, say "no thanks" to the program that your neighbor, your fellow parents, even your therapist suggests. It's not about being paranoid or cynical—it's about being levelheaded and responsible. Do you really want to subject your child to this? Can this really benefit him? Does it address a specific, existing issue in your child where other measures may have failed? Does it make sense to you that this would work? Does it make sense that this would work on the massive scale that the program claims success for?   Trust your intuition—and use your brain. If you still aren't sure about it, you may want to contact a trusted, respected doctor, fellow parent, therapist, consultant, or other professional or friend who should not make the decision for you, but can help you walk through the critical thinking steps to help you make the right choice. Understand that if there were already a true cure for autism, it would have made the cover of *Time* magazine by now, and there would not be any need to advertise via a weird collection of cryptic, high-energy testimonials on a vague website. If there were a single, specific program that universally transformed the performance of all children with autism into the typical, everyday kids you see in the mainstream, it would not be absent from the mention of your doctor, your teacher, your therapists, and the Autism Society of America, or this very book as I write it, all of whom and which have professional experience with autism and what it really means in your child's life. The truth is, there is no single "thing" that will "cure" or "transform" your child right now. It's a combination of things—your own efforts included—that *will* bring your child to a place of optimal, personal success and independence. Nobody has yet bottled, branded, or invented it. And if they try to make you think they have, I'd look closely at what's at stake and what you may be in for, including false hopes and the dissipation of a dream (not to mention needlessly parting you from your hard-earned dollars), and make a choice that puts mind over make-believe. We all wish they weren't out there doing things like this to target you and your child.

But they are, so you need to make choices accordingly.

11) **Take Responsibility: Don't Blame Autism.** This is one of the most critical concepts in autism intervention, period. Master this, and you stand a wonderful chance at being a great positive influence in the life of someone with autism. One of the most common questions I am asked on radio shows, in interviews, and in passing by other professionals is, "What do you do that makes your work so effective? What do you do know that we don't?" The answer, in a nutshell, is very simple, and is not mine alone. I assume first that the person with autism is entirely capable of everything I seek to teach him, and that any weaknesses demonstrated in his performance are due to my own failure to *teach* it in the right way for him. When something doesn't work, I approach it as if it has nothing to do with the person's autism or disability, but rather, with my own "disability" to reach this person effectively. So I put on my thinking cap, get creative, and try something new, because I don't like failing, especially when it comes to failing someone with autism. And here's the most important part of it all-I try this reinventing of my approach, stopping what doesn't help and starting something new, over and over and over again until it works, or until I am 100% sure that I can leave this issue behind without the slightest trace of "what if he could have...." In many, many cases, breakthrough achievements come alive for these individuals with autism once they are finally treated respectfully, and by someone who takes on the full level of serious responsibility that I believe being the parent and/or professional in an autistic child's life merits. In my own standard of professional ethics, if a skill cannot

be mastered by a person with autism, I have to be able to walk away from the situation and look this person's parents, teachers, possibly him or her directly in the eyes and say with 100% sincerity and compassion, "I honestly gave this my best. My personal opinion here is that your child is not likely to develop this skill in the future. I advise taking another course of action, and planning for a set of compensatory skills that will achieve the closest results towards independence, while fostering fulfillment and happiness for this individual. This is not a dead end, but a new beginning on a different course of action! I am tapped out of ideas and options for this specific goal, but I am simply one human being who has done my best. You may always seek to continue where I left off if your gut feeling is different from mine and tells you there is more to try. But I offer you my experience and caring guidance to move forward in a new direction that is realistic, positive, and helpful. Now, let's get to work on an alternate plan or set of options!" I refrain from using the words "will never" or "cannot." Can anyone really say for sure that she/he knows the limits to the capability that lies within someone with autism? Are there truly limits to human capability? I don't dare pretend to have that level of knowledge, and I'd run quickly from anybody who speaks as if his opinion is the only opinion out there! For your benefit and the benefit of all those who stand to reap the value of it, I will reframe this concept here for you:

Always assume first that someone with autism *can* do it, and that it is your responsibility to bring out the success that is buried within him. Pretend you've been gifted with a fistful of seeds, and you don't know which ones

are viable and which are infertile. Make it your job to
plant them all, to try them all, until you see that flower
of success bloom from within. If and when you have
tried all of your seeds, and nothing grows there, then
acquire a special new seed that *will* grow in the soil and
climate of your autistic friend's existing heart,
capabilities, and inner resources. Then marvel at this
creative new bloom, the one that sets the beauty of his
soul in motion, and that brings success into the daylight.
In doing this, you can never fail, and you will never fail
a friend with autism.

The truth is, we see inability and disability all the time.
We look it straight in the eyes, we accept it, we embrace
it. We sigh, "My child has autism. He will never do
this or that," or, "My student isn't able to do so and
so, but that's okay." We need to be able to accept
disabilities of all kinds if we are to be a productive
society! When one person in a marriage is terrible with
finances, the other will organize bills and file taxes. And
the partner who is not financially savvy will contribute
in other ways: she/he will bring income to the
household's bottom line, or take the cars for oil changes,
or know how to soothe a child with a skinned knee.
In society, we readily accept our own limitations and
capabilities, and we define our lives in such a way
that the limitations are minimized and the capabilities
maximized. The problem with most autism intervention
today is not a lack of understanding for the limitations
or disability of people with autism—it's a lack of
understanding for the *ability* of people with autism.
Fine, so your son cannot do this. But can he do that?
Your student cannot write an essay, but can she give you
an oral report? Your daughter cannot go to college, but

can she attend an adult social skills group, learn select subjects from a tutor, or volunteer at the local animal shelter? Your 36-year-old brother with autism cannot interact with customers at the store face to face, but can he break down and stack boxes in the warehouse of the store, write publicity literature and design graphics for the website, or conduct inventory during hours when customers are not shopping? Assume first that your child with autism can do it. If you are eventually proven wrong, know that you are then on the most proven, appropriate path to discover what she/he *can* do. Autism intervention is not about identifying things that people cannot do and coping with it—it's about opening doors to what they *can* do and thriving with it. Being a great autism professional or parent, then, is about being the person who opens those doors. You cannot walk through them for any child, with or without autism. But you can open them. It won't happen by shoving all of your potential for success onto someone else, like your students or children with autism. And it won't happen by blaming circumstances or labels like autism, disability, income, resources, time, even knowledge. It will happen when you step up to the plate and say, "I'm going in here! I'm bringing my best energy, knowledge, and efforts to the table, and I will not stop until I know with 100% of my being that there is no more that I can do. It's not about identifying limits or abilities in someone with autism. It's about identifying my own limits and abilities. When I look at it this way, I can assure everyone involved that this child is getting my absolute best. I am going to make a difference here, and the only question is, how much of a difference?"

In Judaism, there is a very remarkable story of a non-Jew coming to Rabbi Hillel, an ancient sage, and asking if Hillel would teach him the whole Torah (Bible) while standing on one foot. Can you imagine a question like this, asking if all of your wisdom in an entire religion could be reduced to what is learned while standing on one foot?! Hillel replied, "What is despicable to you, do not do unto your neighbor. The rest is commentary. Now go and learn!" Essentially, the lesson was simple— The Golden Rule is what matters most. In the world of autism, The Golden Rule still applies, and this chapter is perhaps "The Golden Rule" of autism intervention. It means, don't just pawn off your own shortcomings and blame them on someone else's autism. If you stood on one foot to hear it, I'd simply say, treat your neighbors with autism kindly, and do so with all of your heart and hard work! The rest, my friends, is commentary—now go and learn!

12) **Stop Micromanaging.** Remember that old boss you used to have, the one who would stand over your shoulder, watching what you were doing, and give "constructive criticisms" to "help" you be more "efficient" on the job? This boss was so "good at his job" and "on top of things" with you that you never had a chance to shine your brightest, because he was always overshadowing you, cutting you off with his "suggestions" before you had the chance to demonstrate that you could have done it perfectly on your own! You couldn't stand that guy, so why would you *become* that guy when it comes to a child's learning process? If you're like most parents and teachers, you know it's important to provide the proper support to students with autism so that they are not left floundering in an academic sea of confusion that

was never designed with them in mind. So you may be surprised to learn that sometimes, the worst thing a parent or teacher can do to hinder a child's forward progress is to suffocate his opportunities to learn and practice independence! This happens all day long in formidable, otherwise well run and appropriately outfitted classrooms across the globe, and I am on a personal mission to stop it, and fast! Why? Because just like every other person on the planet, someone with autism must master a skill independently in order for it to be a true, useable skill. And perhaps most significantly, in more cases than not, when the proper teaching approach and supports are in place, people with autism *can* do things independently when they are aligned with their abilities! Think about it—at some point, your parents eventually took the training wheels off of your bike, right? They stopped reading stories to you, and started letting you read stories to them, even if you mispronounced some words along the way. What to order in a restaurant was no longer decided by mom and dad, but left in your capable hands: "The menu is right there, choose something. You know what you like!" At school, your academic independence was fostered primarily through the administration of those dreaded things called "tests." In order to assess what you had mastered academically, teachers gave you an opportunity to present your knowledge and skills *without any support or interference from anyone else.* Torturous as the process may or may not have been for some of us, it effectively created space for children to demonstrate personal abilities and weaknesses. Weaknesses that were identified through testing were then accurately identified and addressed. But far too often for our students with autism, something else entirely is happening. Loving, caring, intelligent, and qualified teachers and parents are wrongly presumptuous in their approach to autism, assuming that their valiant, extra-attentive, even overprotective efforts will lead a child to success. Not true! Prepare yourself, here—this is a very important concept. *It is the individual with autism's efforts that will ultimately lead to personal success, and it is simply your job as a parent or professional to create every opportunity imaginable for that success!* This is why meaningful motivators, proper environment, and appropriate teaching styles are so critical: not so that we can credit ourselves with the successes of our loved ones with autism, but so that we can foster, inspire, and develop these successes from within them!

The goal of every parent and professional working with an individual with autism should be to create a life of maximum independence for the person with autism, just as our parents attempted to do for us! And just like all the rest of us out there, people with autism operate and function at various different levels of independence. Quick: think of a friend you know who is totally codependent when it comes to relationships, and can't stand being single even for a few months. Now think of another friend, one who can't commit to anyone and isn't in any kind of hurry to "settle down." Both are your friends, and both demonstrate "typical" human behaviors in the sense that this type of behavioral pattern can be routinely found everywhere! The similarities in broad functioning you'll find in those with autism are significant and noteworthy, as are the differences. One critical difference in our two "typical" friends and our autistic friends is that with autism, many individuals will not naturally evolve over time into a state of personal independence. Consequently, there is a much greater emphasis put on the roles that others play in their lives versus the roles that they play in their *own* lives. This is such a detriment! Upon hearing this, many people develop a scowl or weird expression on their faces akin to the thought, "are you nuts, lady? My child with autism is severely impaired, and he can't do much on his own, and what he can do won't make a difference in the long run because he's still going to require supervision and support throughout his life! So why not just make it easier on him and keep him happy? You must not be talking to me—this must be about "high functioning" people with autism, right?" Nope. It's about all of us, and all of our friends with autism. Happiness for someone with autism can be framed just as your happiness was by your parents when you were young. You were allowed to make decisions and lead the way with your own preferences and abilities—to a point. You might choose to swim instead of go play Frisbee with your friends, and that was fine. But if you wanted to stay in that freezing cold swimming pool for too long, remember that your mom would yank you right out of that pool, purple lips and all! You were not empowered to make every decision in your life, but you were empowered to make the ones that were appropriate to your personal level of maturity, wisdom, and ability. You want a hamburger for lunch, fine! You want a super-sized banana split to yourself for dessert when you're five years old but not today! Good, solid autism intervention decreases your child's dependency on others, and capitalizes upon his or her maturity, wisdom, and ability, however unique, limited, or astounding it may be. This is especially noteworthy for our friends with Asperger's Syndrome, who might, say, be able to attend collegiate level courses in a certain area of interest well before reaching middle-school age. However unusual and atypical that would be for a "regular" kid without AS, it *can* be appropriate for *your* child with AS. But while a typical classmate might be able to make the independent choice on how to tell a classmate that he can't come over to play this weekend, your child might need help phrasing this politely so as not to come across as unappreciative of the invitation. All of this is okay! Independence is critical—and very much individually based.

Here's a perfect example of why independence matters regardless of where your child's current performance is. A child who is nonverbal, autistic, and also diagnosed with limited intellectual abilities may be working in school to learn the names of his classmates. With his classmates Tom, Gina, and Rachel standing in front of him, the teacher says, "Who is Tom?" The student with autism remains still and expressionless, and the teacher promptly points and says "*He* is Tom!" She then asks the question again, "Who is Tom?" and repeats the process, satisfied that her autistic student is learning appropriately. Now I have a question for the teacher: how do you know that your student would not have answered properly by himself if you'd simply allotted him a moment of extra time to process (since he has a *processing* disorder known as autism)? Wouldn't this have been a greater achievement, reflecting higher success for both your student and your level of competency as a teacher? Moreover, have you noticed that you are giving yourself a lesson more so than your

student with autism?! Who is this benefiting, anyhow?
I encourage the "Seven Second Rule" to be applied
here: give children with autism a very full seven second
count before intervening with an answer yourself. This
means mentally counting to yourself: "one-one-
thousand, two-one-thousand, three-one-thousand," and
so forth. Maybe he won't come up with an answer, but
maybe he will.

What this all boils down to is to stop unnecessarily
prompting people with autism so much! If someone
truly needs the prompting, that will be evident at some
point. But we cannot assume that people with autism—
and yes, that includes adults with autism spectrum
disorders as well as children—constantly need our
prompting in order to function at their most basic
levels of independence. Of course, they need your
help and support and prompting in many areas. But
they do not need your prompting in *all* areas! Aside
from when you are specifically employing errorless
learning techniques, there is just no good reason to
interrupt potential for independence with co-dependent
behaviors on the part of the parent or teacher! If you
are working on handwriting samples with your student,
once you have a good baseline sense of her capabilities,
please, do not sit right next to her or hover over her
shoulder "watching" her complete a handwriting
worksheet! Move to another area and busy yourself with
something else. If your student's work ultimately shows
that she can do it, won't you feel glad that you didn't
micromanage her to death and leave everybody—
yourself, your student, and her parents—wondering if
she can "really" do this on her own? Great job—that's
really teaching! If you come back and your student has

made chaos on paper with her pencil, then you can require a higher quality of work in a "redo" that reflects her proven ability in writing to replace the garbage she just tried to turn in. Hey, we've all tried to get away with things like this at one time or another in childhood! Try not to make everything a child does exclusively a characteristic of autism. You certainly don't want to minimize the very real effects of autism in your student's life, but try to remember that sometimes, a kid is just being a kid! Otherwise, you've potentially taught your student the wrong things! Do you want to set her up to believe that sub-standard work is okay, even when it's below her reasonable abilities and will not get her by when she tries to apply it in the real world? Do you want her to think that she's only obligated to concentrate or work when someone is watching, enforcing, supervising her? Think of it this way—is it practical, useful, or even purposeful to teach a child to perform only under the watchful eye of an adult? Not really. Can you be more effective by removing your influence and instead, allowing the child to perform without your hovering presence? Absolutely! This is called *generalizing* a skill, and it's actually just as important to your child's future as getting the basic concept of the skill itself. After all, what happens when this student leaves your classroom for good, and the new teacher does not behave in the exact same way that you did? If the skill that you allegedly "taught" your autistic student can't hold up in another classroom or in a similar real-world environment without your influence, then it wasn't really "taught" properly to begin with. It just doesn't matter how beautiful her handwriting is "with you," if she won't write that way anywhere else. It's not a triumph or testimony to your great teaching—it means that you missed a few critical steps, and you need to go back and do a more comprehensive teaching job! It doesn't matter if you can brag that your son's table manners are sublime at home. If he's throwing stuff on the floor and spilling his juice onto his peas to see if they float at a playmate's house, then you've got some work to do, and a reality check to help you do it!

You must remember to always apply one of the most commonly heard, and commonly undervalued phrases in education today—*least restrictive* measures. We hear this so often used in a legal context for special education, but not often enough when it comes to actual, specific approaches to individual learning tasks. *Least restrictive* as a concept is so much more than a legal parameter at school—it is the best practice for all of your approaches to educating someone with autism at school, at home, and everywhere. Too often, I meet parents and teachers who *think* they know, understand, and utilize least restrictive measures for their students with autism. Instead, I find a lot of least restrictive placement in education, but not practical, everyday classroom applications of the idea for specific academic lessons, behavioral management, or other direct service areas. Least restrictive education means affording your child the supports she/he truly needs to help compensate for potential deficits or special needs, but no more than what is truly required and needed! Lots of people misread this notion as a negative one, fearing that additional supports and efforts that could potentially benefit a child are deliberately, even coldly, withheld because it's not legally required. They think "least restrictive" is a term that benefits the schools, and the accounts that the schools are keeping. Nothing could be further from the truth! What least restrictive can mean and is designed to foster is that your child has maximum access to supports that are necessary, and that unnecessary accommodations that might make your child stand out more, become dependent upon something unnecessary, or otherwise compromise your child's true level of independent performance will not be introduced. How does least restrictive education work in action? It's simple. Let's say your child is having a whole lot of trouble with keeping his hands to himself during walks in the hallway between classrooms. He's touching everything, maybe even touching everyone, holding up the line, pulling down artwork that's hanging in front of classrooms, and generally, not succeeding to be appropriately independent and self-controlled. How does a teacher commonly respond to this dilemma? She/he disciplines the student for poor conduct or behavior, and probably holds his hand at the front of the line, or has a teaching assistant hold his hand or monitor him closely by walking alongside him. The behavior is consequently eliminated! Good job, problem solved, right? Maybe, maybe not. Let's think about this from a more generalized perspective. Now we have a student who has been disciplined for what was wrong, and contained by physical redirection so that he's not able to do it again under those circumstances. But what if you let go of the child's hand, and look the other way, or have a substitute present to lead the students? Does he still have the freedom and tools for success to make it down the hallway appropriately? I don't know, but probably not. How old is this student? If his peers are able to walk down the hallway without holding the teacher's hand, then it probably makes him stand out as needing much more support and being a "baby" in front of his friends. It may or may not be embarrassing to the student himself. Also, he now knows what *not* to do, but is there something he knows he *can* do instead to self-manage his touchy-feely urges? Hmm—I'm afraid not. Then there is the issue of generalization. Is this student now equipped to manage this behavior not just under the direct supervision of this one teacher in this one specific scenario, but for *all* of his walks down school and other hallways for all of his life in any other kind of class or building? Unfortunately, nobody has taken the time to consider these real-world issues, and while the teacher and parent of this particular student may feel great now and have a temporary sense of security that this behavior is gone, that security is probably false, and the behavior will probably rear its head again. But what if we take this same situation and approach it from a least-restrictive angle?

Instead of the above "solution," a truly comprehensive least restrictive approach would eliminate all of the "restrictive" aspects of this situation. I'd add an extra classroom "job" to our job chart and assign the job, "Teaching Materials Assistant," to the young man. I'd give this student a stack of my books to carry that "need" to be transported from our original classroom to the next destination. They would be just heavy enough to require both arms and both hands, but not so heavy that the student needs to put them down or struggles to carry them. I'd leave the student alone, and let him stand wherever he would naturally place in line each day. It's a replacement behavior that is incompatible with touching others or pulling artwork off of the walls. It builds his self-esteem and rewards independence, rather than disciplines him for something negative and restricting him to depend on a teacher's physical redirection! Instead of standing out as being needy or childish in the eyes of his peers, he's seen as fitting in more by doing an assigned job just as they all do. This same method could be easily applied in any hallway, by any teacher or parent, in any building, and best of all, teaches the student what he *can* do instead of touching others and grabbing at artwork! This skill is easily generalized to all other environments, where the boy can come prepared with his own stack of "materials" in hand to help him keep his hands where they are appropriate. Voila! This is the beauty and splendor of least restrictive education! You could achieve the same results with creating a "hands in pockets" rule for the whole class so no student is singled out (but you've got to make sure children have pockets in their clothing, as in school uniforms, or otherwise you might topple this idea and go for something else instead). Hopefully you now understand why I strongly prefer you to refrain from hovering over your student as she does her handwriting: it's not least restrictive and it's not productive! By applying least restrictive measures to every approach you take with an autistic child or adult, you are not clipping their wings—you are teaching them to soar!

13) **Stop and Smell the Roses**—and the garlic in your spaghetti sauce, and the bleach in the rags used to wipe down tables at school, and the gaudy, sugary-sweet perfume your son's teacher wears! Realize that it's a whole different world out there to people with autism who experience life with over-developed senses, or

under-developed senses. Imagine this: what's the worst smell you can think of—sewage, rotten milk, body odor, vile garbage? Does it make you frown, gag, feel nauseated, stay back? Now imagine what life would be like if your workplace had a room that smelled pungently of that odor and you were expected to walk in there, work diligently, communicate effectively without distraction, and even eat your lunch alongside that hideous smell? It seems unimaginable to us, yet we send our children with autism into these scenarios daily, and grossly underestimate the kind of impact that those five senses we learned all about in kindergarten *really* have on our kids. We often focus on sensory integration for children with autism, but we do not often enough consciously think about the *reason* that sensory integration came into being, or why it is important to generalize the concept of sensory integration to more than a type of therapy involving those more common OT activities! Mentally go through your senses right now: hearing, touch, taste, smell, and sight. If you were Superman or Superwoman, and your senses were extra-sensitive, what kinds of things might you notice about your home, your car, your child's classrooms, even the people and objects your child comes in contact with daily? This is not to say you should become paranoid, modifying and sterilizing your child's environments so that they are no longer a real-world experience. It is an opportunity to see, touch, taste, smell, and feel the world through your child's senses, and to respond with actions that make that world more negotiable for him. Do you love to dress your little girl in frilly, girly, adorable dresses because they look so cute on her? Many parents like to dress their autistic children adorably, because they feel it helps their kids fit in better if they are look sharp. Maybe so! But not if your little girl makes a spectacle of herself in kindergarten every time she peels her cute white tights off and drops them under the table, or spends half of class scratching at the ruffles and lace that scrape at her chest and belly through her dress. Are you getting reports that she was "extra wiggly" today, or "squirming a lot in her seat"? Examine why—and fire your internal wardrobe consultant if necessary! By thinking through your child's current environmental through the eyes of a super-charged sensory system, you can empower yourself with critical wisdom about *why* your child behaves the way she does in many cases. Is she chewing, gnawing, pinching, hitting, or showing other physical signs of sensory needs? Is she tugging at, covering, plugging, or scratching at her ears? Give her what she needs in a socially-appropriate, independent, manageable way.

Beyond the built-in standards of swinging, jumping, and spinning that can be fundamentally useful (and fun) for kids with autism in need of physical outlets, empower your child with small, personal intervention tools to help her cope with sensory differences. Provide gum, a chewy tube, a lollipop, or other foods or items to help alleviate jaw stress, chewing, grinding, gnawing, and biting. The "Livestrong" rubber bracelets that are made as a cancer fundraiser come in a child size, and they are just as tough and chewy as a chewy tube, but "look cool" and fit in with today's trends! Think about texture (does she relax with soft foods to eat, and tense up for crunchy things?), temperature (could a juice pop help her, or would she prefer a warm cup of cocoa?), and density (does she like to bite "chewy" things like skin and rubber, hard things like desk corners and textbooks, or soft things like sweaters and shirts?). Dress her in heavier, lighter, or softer clothing to help calm squirming, wiggling, scratching, and rubbing up against items. Think about textures and pressures for those issues, like a wool coat versus cotton, a light windbreaker (which also makes a distracting "swish" sound with movement) versus a heavier leather jacket.

Make sure her hearing is addressed. It's the most likely sensory issue to be bothering her. Is there a noise coming from the computer monitor that distracts her? Seat her away from it! Is the intercom system emitting a high-pitched hum, or the child seated behind yours fidgeting with pencils in her desk cubby, making a clicking sound? Is her neighbor stuffed up with a cold, and breathing heavily through his mouth? Pay attention and do what you can to help her focus. Visually, do the flickering fluorescent lights keep her from focusing? Are there way too many colorful distractions on the walls, or not enough visual supports to help her follow the flow of class? Provide a stress ball to squeeze, a stamp pad, sturdy rubber stamp, and paper to apply pressure to, or mini hand exercisers to squeeze to help meet the proprioceptive needs as an alternative to hitting for input. The stamp pad is a great way to help manage that need some children feel to "whack" or "bang" things. Ask the teacher to make your child his helper for "grading" papers, and have her stamp the class assignments regularly! Now here's where I want you to be careful—sensory issues are a part of autism, but they are only *one* part of autism! Try not to jump on the sensory bandwagon to the extent that you forget about the other major obstacles your child contends with that are *not* necessarily related to sensory needs at all. If your child is verbal, but is struggling with receptive language skills, don't just write it off as a sensory problem within the classroom. That's a *part* of your child's autism, not something the classroom has created!

14) **Form an Entourage.** Okay, so he's not a celebrity. But your child with autism needs an entourage of top-notch special needs professionals who can acutely and comprehensively address his overall needs. In addition to your role as a magnificent parent, you may need to enlist the services of a diagnostician, special educators, regular educators, support specialists, speech and occupational therapists, a psychiatrist for medications, a consultant or advocate to help design a great educational or intervention plan and ensure that effective goals are in place and operating, a babysitter and/or respite service who knows your child so that you can still take moments off to live your own life, a neighbor, fellow special needs parent, or nearby friend who can serve as an outlet for quick saves when you need to leave in an emergency or can't make it to carpool, and even more. Whew—it's a long list and it isn't even entirely representative of all the possibilities! If you are feeling overwhelmed by these choices or are unsure who to turn to for reliable, autism-savvy services in your area, your best bet might be to contact a few members at your closest ASA group. Often, the ASA groups are equipped with the names and contact information of experienced, preferred professionals in the community. Essentially, if you are regularly surrounding your child with positive, experienced, and effective autism professionals, you

are increasing his interaction with people who can make a difference in his life just by being around!

15) **Buy a megaphone.** This, of course, is only necessary if you cannot speak up. So the real message is: *speak up!* Speak up at your child's IEP, at your child's therapy offices, at your child's boy scout troop, and everywhere else where your voice can make a difference in the experiences of your child. Speaking up is not being pushy, being demanding, or being antagonistic. It is simply *bringing the positive contributions that you can add to your child's daily existence to the attention of those who are in a position to help.* There is no place for the timid in special education! If you are timid, then you may consider hiring a professional advocate to "be" your voice for you.

16) **Use What Works.** Not everything in autism intervention has to be an uphill battle. Instead of focusing extra-heavily on experimental and/or unconfirmed interventions (this does not mean to avoid these things entirely), make sure that the biggest chunk of your child's intervention is based in what has already proven to work. You do not have to reinvent the wheel when it comes to behavioral and educational approaches to autism, for example. You should realize that a lot of what's out there in the autism community today can be considered "experimental" or "alternative" simply because barely any concrete medical research has been done to confirm or deny that effectiveness of such interventions. For this reason, I cannot suggest that you avoid them, fear them, or reject them, nor can I suggest that they are worth your energy, efforts, dollars, hopes, and time. Even therapies and approaches that we might

consider as generally "accepted" in the autism community, such as certain sensory and auditory training approaches, come with little data for verification. This does not necessarily mean that you cannot or should not consider trying these therapies. Biomedical and dietary interventions are also widely popular and commonplace today, and although there is little mainstream data and scientific research devoted to advocating these approaches, you may find the information you need to make an informed choice by talking to other parents, professionals, and by reading up on the myriad of organized resources online. There's no need to exclude or include any therapy simply based on someone else's opinion, but perhaps in future years we will have sufficient and concrete data to help us make medically-sound and ethically-sound choices about the programs we employ for our children with autism.

In the meantime, the best approach to employ for your child's intervention is to create a reasonable program that, tailored to your child's needs and your personal beliefs, is much more heavily focused on proven intervention, and lightly focused on experimental intervention. By relying too heavily on the experimental side, you run the risk of finding out that, in the end, these things did not work for your child and precious intervention time was lost forever. On the other hand, trying experimental interventions—provided that they are safe, medically supervised by qualified, accredited professionals in their field (OT, medicine, etc.)—can open up the possibility for your child to benefit from something that may later be proven effective. And what's been proven effective for children with autism now? Well, depending upon the child's individual needs, there is data to support the TEACCH methodology (a wonderful approach, and one that I both recommend and incorporate widely into my own best practices), Applied Behavior Analysis or ABA (the greatest amount of research data exists on the effectiveness of these techniques, which can be useful either in strict accordance with ABA standards or in varying contexts using the core concepts), Occupational Therapy, Speech Therapy, and to some extent, research is emerging on programs such as Floortime. The list of accepted and/or existing resources for autism intervention is way too long to list here. But know that your child is most likely to build achievements based on existing methods that have been proven to lead to success. However, it is important to note that just because an approach or program has not been researched and outlined as "officially" effective does not necessarily make it bad or unethical. But it could be, so use your best judgment when subjecting your child to any therapeutic intervention for any reason, from any source.

17) **Be Creative.** It's important to use what's already out there; what's already available for your child in the way of effective, meaningful techniques, programs, resources, and concepts. To effectively "use what works," you do not need to reinvent the wheel when approaching your child's autism intervention. By the same token, you do not need to cut off your nose to spite your face, either. If something new, different, or unconventional might help your child where existing resources have failed, then it's time to try it! Don't be afraid to do something on your child's or student's behalf simply because you made it

up. Consider that every single preferred, respected,
reputable, and widely prescribed method of autism
intervention was once nothing more than somebody
else's made-up idea! That's right: some years ago, the
concept and structure of "ABA" was nothing more than
a fresh idea that bounced around loosely in one human
being's mind. What separates the successful ideas and
concepts from the ones that never get implemented? At
least one primary thing: the willingness of people just
like you to explore their ideas through action. We have
so much bloated jargon intimidating parents in the
world of autism. Things aren't "great ideas" anymore,
they're "methodologies." It's not a "teaching style," it's
an "intervention, technique, or development exercise."
We no longer ask "how did you potty train your child,"
but "what toilet training technique or school of thought
do you subscribe to?" And it's not considered standard
to simply refer to your child's daily regimen as
"preschool, extracurricular activities, and play," but
"behavioral intervention program, therapeutic
appointments, and social skills and interactive
development sessions." Try to remember that in the
thick of all this, your child is still a child, and you are
still a parent—no lofty terminology can change that!
Focus less on what things are called, which brand name
it most closely resembles or doesn't, or what your idea
would be "classified" as, and just do it! There does not
need to be any foundation to your idea beyond this: you
believe it might work, you understand it's safe and
reasonable, and you can maintain your sense of humor if
it doesn't yield results. If you've got this creative idea to
teach your child how to hold a spoon by dangling one
from the ceiling, having him "grab" it, and "race" to

scoop up oatmeal against his dad and older brother, then go ahead—the Methodology Police might not make it to your neighborhood tonight! To be a great, wonderful parent to a child with autism, sometimes we just need to relax about all the information buzzing around us, and make up something new. Chances are that some fragments of effective methodology will be buried within your creation anyhow, because good ideas usually come to more than one person at a time! This is true not only about autism intervention, but in life—the best ideas are widely recycled in the minds of many. In the case of "oatmeal racing," for example, you've got a hint of mirroring peers in there, a dash of assistive equipment (e.g., the string you use to hang the spoon, which supports it and makes it easier for your child to grab without dropping), and a therapeutic play aspect which can double as a motivator! Of course, you also run the risk of stumbling upon a real humdinger there. Hello, does anyone else remember the piano necktie? Some things just aren't meant to last. But then again, if the inventor of that tie did so to captivate the interest of and teach his autistic savant son, who was a musical genius on the piano, how to properly knot his tie, then I revoke my previous statement and think it's a great idea! Go ahead—make things up as you go along. Successful autism intervention is 1/3 knowledge, 1/3 hard work, and 1/3 creativity!

18) **Make Final Plans.** It is never too early to plan for your child's future beyond the years that you will be there to care for her. Parents often ask me, "When is the ideal time to start planning for my child's care for after I'm gone?" The answer is that if your child has received a diagnosis, it's time to start planning. Don't assume that

the state will kick in funds to help out. Don't assume a relative will pass away and leave you a large inheritance. Don't assume that if you could just cover your current expenses, you'd save more when you get a better job, a smaller house, a bigger raise. Start planning and saving now. To clarify, I mean today, or preferably, yesterday! The best way to do this is to research the projected costs for the level of care that your child will need, whether residential, supported living, or even just renting an apartment. Think about day services, hiring a job coach, hiring someone to help do grocery shopping, laundry—whatever level of help your child will need as an adult. Get on waiting lists as early as the programs in question will allow. Visit them, explore them, meet people. Talk to parents who have adult children with autism, and ask them to guide you through what they're doing for their child, how it's working, and what they would have done differently. Don't wait until it's three years before your child needs to leave home for services, and don't put it off because you think it might be upsetting or depressing. The peace of mind that comes from knowing that your child is taken care of, no matter what, will likely be a priceless asset to your loving heart. By the time your child is a young teenager or earlier, start figuring out what programs are available, what the costs are, how program content, philosophies, and costs compare. By that age, you'll have a pretty good feel for the degree of long-term services your child will require. Prior to the middle school and teen years, I recommend that you save as if your child will require the most extensive and expensive services out there. That way, you are prepared for that *and* anything less than that.

19) **Ask For Help.** Quit trying to be Superwoman and
Superman, parents. When you need help—with how to
address a behavior, how to teach tying shoelaces, or how
to prepare dinner without seeing your child running
naked around the living room with a crayon in his
nose and a pair of your pantyhose hanging out the back
of his diaper. *Ask someone.* When you just need your
own time alone, ask for help. When you as parents need
time together, ask for help. If you need to fund an
important intervention and don't know if you'll be able
to do so alone, ask for help. And if you're like most
parents of children with autism, you're thinking,
"Hmm—sounds wonderful! Just who is this 'Help'
character?" I'm so glad you asked—I'm happy to help!
Help can come in many forms, some of which you may
already be familiar with, and others that are new to
you. Help can come in the form of a person who lends a
hand, a bit of advice, or a bit of time. A neighbor,
friend, teacher, family member, doctor, therapist,
another special needs parent—they are all sources of
help. Other sources of help can be groups, businesses,
or organizations. You probably realize that your local
Autism Society of America chapter is going to be
mentioned in here somewhere (right here). Although it
sounds clichéd in this autism world, the ASA nearest
you can offer a lot of help, and it's *not* all just in the
form of information packets or support group meetings
where people sit in a circle and go around saying "Hi,
my name is Jennifer and my child has autism!" ASA
chapters frequently have the most valued and respected
local autism professionals visit and speak as guests.
You might just find the best child neurologist, speech
therapist, or even babysitter at an ASA meeting! You

might meet six other moms who have children with autism in your school, and learn which teacher is known for being wonderful with autistic children. You might find free childcare, small support grants, or other treasured resources.

The ASA is not the only organization that can help you, and some might be different than you'd expect. Have you considered the bank as a place to ask for help? If your child's private autism school program is costing an arm and a leg—but is worth it—and your non-autistic daughter just announced her acceptance to Harvard Law School, and your anticipated promotion to Vice President got passed over, you might consider help in the form of financial breathing room. Synagogues, churches, mosques, and other religious communities can often provide lots of special, handy help that really comes from the heart. Congregation volunteers might help with babysitting, carpooling, even yard work if you're strapped for cash or just don't have time. They can also help raise funds to help pay for special therapies, private educational intervention, and medical or pharmaceutical costs. Regardless of your household income, autism intervention is, generally, costly and can impact your family's bottom line. Nobody thinks of it as "charity" or "giving to the poor" when helping to raise funds to cover the costs of medical care and/or therapeutic care for someone in the community. They just think of it as an opportunity to help out, make a difference, and feel good about themselves along the way. So in the end, remember that it's okay to ask for help. It's good to ask for help. And you don't need to be a superhero and do it on your own. To your child, you are already heroes.

20) **Pull That Stick Out of the Mud.** So your bright-eyed three-year-old son with PDD: NOS just poured his glass of milk down his pants to see how it feels. Your precocious eleven-year-old Asperger's daughter, a legend in her own time for crossing social boundaries, just told the woman behind you in the grocery store that her hair looks like "Medusa, a pivotal character in mythological literature." And then, as if things weren't bad enough, your spouse will be coming home late this evening! Do you flip out? Do you shudder in horror? Do you resign yourself to the chaotic and mischievous nature of our cruel world? Or do you *laugh*? If you answered anything other than "laugh," know that this puts you alongside the vast majority of special needs parents— and that's okay! But there is a better way to go about the daily trials and tribulations of life with autism in the mix. Laugh at it! What's that? "It's not funny," you say? Oh, I beg to differ! Consider that some of the most disastrous social and situational happenings seem very serious as they happen—and *very* funny later. Remember those terrible dates your old roommate used to set you up on in college? Think about it—how did you feel during dinner when stuck at a Chinese restaurant splitting greasy veggie lo mein with that cheap guy who wouldn't talk about anything but sword fighting, muscle cars, and Dungeons & Dragons (and then—egads—tried to kiss you at your dorm room door)? Not funny then. Very funny now. What about the time when you went out with a really attractive girl you'd had your eye on all semester and she turned out to be a brainless lush who puked all over your car dash (and you had to spend your Sunday morning trying to

clean her vomit out of the air conditioning vent with Q-tips)? Not funny then. Very funny now. No, I wasn't spying on you in college—these things are relatively universal!

Autism is not any different than any other life event when it comes to learning how to deflect stress, tension, and even flat-out disgust over the things that make us cringe. The trick is, you've got to learn to see the humor in situations *now* instead of *later*! After all, witnessing our children embarrassing us is universal to parents of all children, with or without any type of diagnosis. And most of us have already survived the karmic payback—think about how embarrassed you were about your parents when you were in middle school! Okay, so the things a child with autism does that embarrass you might not be the same things a typical child does to embarrass her parents. But the feelings the parents have *are* pretty similar! Let's face it: you're not going to hitch a ride in a time machine anytime soon to go back and undo the milk in your kid's jeans, or the embarrassing comment made to a stranger at the supermarket. It happened. It was not cool. But it's over. So instead of waiting ten years to laugh about it, just laugh about it now! If you can tell yourself "this is not funny now, but it'll be funny years from now," then simply *allow yourself* to feel the humor in it now. When your child does something cute that's attributed to his autism, you allow yourself to enjoy that moment and laugh at it, right? Well, why not learn to focus the fun-loving, good-natured human tendency to release stress with laughter on all the autism related happenings in your life? If it sounds good in theory but you're having trouble putting this into practice at first, try this.

When autism mischief rears its head, think to yourself, "How would this have been filmed and scripted in a TV sitcom?" Imagine your favorite comedian playing you, and conjure up the imaginary reaction that she/he might have to this situation. Just letting yourself focus on something else funny will help diffuse the tension of the situation right away! Humor is a great healer. It releases stress, banishes tension, and contributes to the release of endorphins that help you physically and literally *feel* better! Does autism or its associated deviant behaviors have your brain on the fritz? Take two jokes and call me in the morning!

And there you have it. Want to be an autism intervention powerhouse? Use the information here, and you'll be giving your child an unstoppable shot at his or her best potential. To do this, the 20 Key Secrets to being a powerfully positive force in your child's autism intervention, then, are as follows:

1) Know Your Child.

2) Claim Your Power.

3) Motivate Meaningfully.

4) Use Your Voice as a Tool Beyond Words.

5) Know Strengths and Weaknesses.

6) Use Visual Cues.

7) Use Replacement Behaviors and Transition Objects.

8) Eliminate Errors.

9) Use Your Intuition.

10) Use Your Brain.

11) Take Responsibility: Don't Blame Autism.

12) Stop Micromanaging.

13) Experience The World Through Your Child's Senses.

14) Hire Great Professionals To Help You.

15) Speak Up.

16) Use What Works.

17) Be Creative.

18) Make Final Plans.

19) Ask For Help.

20) Laugh.

Some important concrete tips have been given here. However, they are not to be substituted for your own good judgment and critical thinking, but *fused* with your own assessment of their value. Too many resources put too much emphasis on what a given professional knows about autism in general, and not enough emphasis on what we can *all* learn from a parent's under-standing of his or her own child. We need to stop putting the responsibility and power for autism intervention so heavily upon the shoulders of outside professionals, and start returning some of the responsibility and power to the insiders—the parents, who know your own children and are greater resources in your chil-dren's lives than anything or anyone else. By "responsibility," this does not mean adding work for parents that is taken away from professionals. On the contrary, I use "responsibility" in the truest, most basic sense of the word—the role of ownership over acceptable final results.

As professionals, we do not intentionally make your choices for you, nor do we intentionally use the power to choose that is so rightfully yours. But sometimes, you must realize that we are sent some rather significant mixed signals. On one end, we hear parents advocating for their children, working to participate, contribute, and commit to doing all they can to inspire successes for their children. On the other hand, we see you at carpool, overwhelmed, exhausted, just ready for a break and an opportunity for someone else to be in charge for just a moment. We see the looks of worry, of fear, of feeling inadequately prepared to make the kinds of choices that will impact your child's life forever. When your child is screaming and tantruming as he enters the doctor's office, and you don't know if you should hold him down or drag him out and never go back, sometimes, you give us that look. That look is the one that says, "I'm drowning in this decision. My heart just can't take it. Can you do this for me? Should I hold him down, or should I take him out?" And we hesitate. And we think. And in the end, we speak up because we love you. We do what we feel will help you and your child, because we care about you both, saying, "I'd_____if it were me." And then, the thinking is over. The advice is followed, and a good thing and a bad thing have happened all at once. For a good choice has been made, but it has been made in a gray world where there are no "right" or "wrong" choices in general, and in the process, your own parental light has been ever so slightly diminished. It has been diminished not because you accepted valuable, caring, knowledgeable help! It has been diminished because you did not add your own beliefs to this mix, instead, immediately following the directions of someone else in order to numb the overwhelming choice that was really yours. All that needs to change in order for this to be purely a good thing is for parents to take back their responsibility—yes, ownership—over the final decisions that come into their children's lives. Gather our opinions—value them, use them! But do not ever allow them to override your own. If you agree with us, and it's validation you're seeking, then we have successfully worked together to make the best choice for the good of your child. If you are seeking freedom from the responsibility to make the choice itself, and you allow us to think for you, then all the magic and beauty that comes from within a parent—that can in most cases *only* come from within a parent—has been forsaken. And so I urge you, I support you—do not abandon your own brilliant thoughts, feelings, and beliefs here! Join your thoughts with ours, and together, we can move mountains for our children with autism!

Parents, you are the only ones who will be with your child for his or her entire lifetime, or yours. In the end, specific professionals and teachers, who need to do everything within their professional power to improve the quality of life for their students, cannot be expected to single-handedly conquer the challenges and obstacles that your child faces. We do all we can for your children. And then, hopefully based on the success of our work, we move on, or your child moves on, because we are no longer needed in the same way as when you first came to us. And this is a beautiful thing, and the way it is supposed to be. For too long, it seems that the information on how to best think critically, strategize, and navigate the world of autism intervention has been cloaked in a haze of jargon, expertise, and a misguided hierarchy of roles that wrongly places professionals at the top, and parents submissively below them. To help your child reach his or her highest potential, do not allow this crumbling system of unspoken and faulty control to infiltrate your own perceptions. Know that you are the king or queen of your child's autism intervention. Teachers, therapists, professionals—we come to your royal court in roles that change daily, from princes and princesses, to court advisors, warriors, to the royal chefs, spiritual clergy, and even jesters. But we are not dictators, nor should we be seen and valued as such. Those of us who behave in such a way as to make you feel inferior, detached from the process of your child's education, or less capable of making a good choice on your child's behalf—well, I suggest you excommunicate those individuals, and banish them from your intervention kingdom. In the end, they will only brew discord for you and all who work for the good of your child's life. If you can take the wisdom in this book, apply it to your own life and cherish the core concepts that empower you, then you may just find that in the end, your child's autism fairytale may turn out closing with a "happily ever after."

AFFIRMATION: MY CHANCE TO SHINE

My child is the greatest gift to me. And I am the greatest gift to my child. Today, I remember that I possess the power to keep my child moving in a positive direction. My child needs me right now, and this is my chance to shine. How can I help him best? What can I do to serve her needs? I am doing a wonderful job and bringing my child forward in this world!

Today, I have the attitude that leads to success for my child.

Today, I have the know-how that leads to success for my child.

Today, I have the spirit that leads to success for my child.

Today, I have the philosophy that leads to success for my child.

Today, I am a part of my child's success.

Yesterday, I was a part of my child's success.

Tomorrow, I will witness my child's success.

This is my chance to shine, and I embrace it!

CHAPTER SIX

REALISM MEETS INSPIRATION

❤ How to handle the rough spots and challenging realities that face us in the world of autism

❤ Affirmation: Rising Above Challenges

Accept the challenges so that you can feel the exhilaration of victory."
-George S. Patton

Some people grew up with family members who would tell
them, "when life gives you lemons, make lemonade." In my family, lots of inspiration came from my grandparents' survival
through the Holocaust. Singled out as Jewish people in Eastern
Europe during the peak years of anti-semitism, they were mortal-
ly condemned for being different. And once they were liberated
from their wrongful torture and imprisonment, their lives were
forever changed. Freedom, to them, always meant something
different than it does to you and me. It was the living joy that
stood for all that destroyed captivity. Money meant something
different to them than it does to you and me. It meant the ability to eat, have shelter, and clothe their children while protecting
them from danger, should another Holocaust ever plague our
world again. And love meant something different to them than
it means to you and me. It meant being there—however "there"
could be interpreted that day—to instill in their children acceptance for who they are as different. It meant helping all of us learn
to accept and embrace that we are Jewish. And it meant helping
all of us to learn to be proud and comfortable with who we are,
and loving, tolerant, and accepting of others for who they are. To
do anything less, in a way, was perhaps like creating a little, private mental Holocaust for someone else. And so I learned to love
and value everyone—every one of us all—for exactly who we are.
This has, in part, defined my success in the world of autism. And
what I've learned from it may in part now help you to define
yours.

Bad things happen to good people. It's undeniable. The
Holocaust happened to my grandparents. A car wreck can hap-

pen to a vibrant teenager. A hurricane can destroy an entire town in one sweeping hour. Autism can happen to your child.

How should we respond in the face of such unsuspected and uninvited life events? Stand up? Be bold? Move on? Maybe. In fact, yes. That is a part of what we are supposed to do in response to events that change our lives in a single instant. But perhaps the greatest gift that we can give ourselves and our loved ones with autism is not to see the autism as a tragedy at all—not to view it as a "bad" thing that happened to a "good" person. Because viewing autism as "bad" suggests that we must get rid of it from within our children. And believing that—well, that undoes the cherished peace that we have now made with autism. And undoing peace invites the presence of unrest. And unrest leads to pain, confusion, and struggle, which is, in fact, the source of why we need to work towards feeling inner peace! So how do you handle it when you find out that some elements of autism are not that great, are not convenient, and are probably not going to go away?

You handle it in exactly the same manner that you handled the news from your doctor when she told you, "Your child has autism." There's shock. Anger. Sadness. Anger. Frustration. Disbelief. Denial. Anger. And then—acceptance. Before you understood or accepted that your child had autism, nothing much could be done to help him overcome the things he needed to overcome, and to reach the goals he needed to reach. Today, you've already moved mountains to help your child access all the best strategies to help him. You accepted that he has autism, and then, you met the truth with action.

Do not focus on the feeling or judgment your
mind wants to attach to the truth.
Instead, accept the truth, and respond to it with action.

I'm not saying it's easy. And I'm not even saying that I've been there, or that I know how you feel. I haven't, and I don't. Not for this. But we are all a network of human friends, and I promise you, someone else, somewhere else, has already been in your shoes. And most importantly, she/he got past this point, and is working towards a different truth right now. You have the power to move forward at your discretion in the world of autism. If you've ever watched an *Oprah Winfrey Show* where a victim of recent tragedy bears her soulful confusion on TV, then is met by another remarkable woman who has already endured a similar challenge in the past, then you understand what I'm sharing with you now. Your experience—however individual and unique—is still, and will always be connected to the greater human experience. Maybe you realize today the truth that your child will probably always be nonverbal. Maybe today you discover that your son will not one day live on his own. And you might find out that college, marriage, and career options will never be what you once dreamed of for your child. These things will surely weigh on your heart. But do not be so remiss as to let it weigh on your heart without also taking action to *lighten* your spirit. Will your child be nonverbal? Okay! What can you do to put a different communication system in place? Do it! Will your child require support staff into adulthood? Okay! What can you do to arrange this for him? If college, marriage, and career are not options, are creative adult education, friendships, and volunteerism possibilities? Nothing is going to make you "feel better" about a struggle or challenge more than *addressing* the challenge head on! We can work harder and harder, day after day to provide the best autism intervention possible. And still, some efforts will not yield the final results we'd hoped for. We cannot apply quality intervention and say that children who do not speak will be free to speak once they "finish" intervention. We cannot say that those who are unable to read today will surely be able to read tomorrow. But we can—and must—insist that for every possibility, the work is done to achieve the *best result possible for that individual child.*

> *My goal is to improve the quality of life for individuals with autism, one heart at a time.*

It is a goal that never fails me, and it never fails a child or adult friend with autism. I hope it is a goal that you will share with me. Our friends with autism will cherish the work that we do to meet this goal, and they will cherish those who care for them enough to help reach it. They will not begrudge you for "failing" to teach them to read. They will adore you for teaching them to turn on the television set! They will not begrudge you for their remaining nonverbal. They will cherish you for teaching them to sign! They will not love you less for focusing on the things they can do. They will thank you for gracefully letting go of what they cannot do, and for laying the expectations that will not be met, finally, to rest. They will love you for doing your best. And you will love them for doing theirs.

Many people like to talk about those with autism not connecting well with others. But it seems to me that, as you work together to maintain that fine balance of each doing your best for the other, perhaps relationship skills are relative. How many parents of typical children are privy to the honor of *collaborating* with their child on the creation of the child's best quality of life daily? Not everyone has a chance to do so. But you do. You have that chance with your child every day. And it is nothing less than a blessing, and no less significant than a miracle. So when adversity strikes you in the world of autism, keep walking forward. It's a bump in the road, no doubt! But you can get past it. So can your child. It's not a hurricane, a holocaust, a car crash—it's autism. It's an obstacle you did not ask for and did not expect. But you got it, and it's here. There are plenty of things you can do about it. Autism is real, and comes with no cure. It's tough, it's tenacious, and it's in your face every day. But it is treatable, manageable, and livable! So live it—and live it well!

AFFIRMATION:
RISING ABOVE CHALLENGES

I've seen what a fire looks like in my lifetime. I've watched the fire burn, while seeing the smoke curl in graceful wisps, soaring high above its source. I've seen the smoke rise—a product of that raging fire—as if it were floating on the wings of angels. Today, I choose to float above the fire of autism. Today, I choose to rise to the height of angels. Autism is my challenge, and I gracefully rise above it.

I did not ask for autism in my life. But it's here, so I accept it. I did not ask for the challenges that autism presents, but they are here, so I accept them.

What I asked for—a beautiful, wonderful, fantastic child—is also here, and I accept that.

What challenges will autism present today? I do not know yet, but I know that I can handle them! What obstacles will make me stumble and fumble for what to do? I do not know yet, but I know that I can handle them! And what if I do not know how to handle them? It is out of the question, because I have always found a way so far, and today will be no different!

I invite the universe to smooth my experience with autism, and to lessen my obstacles and lighten my challenges. But for those things that must come my way, I am ready!

CHAPTER SEVEN

THE WORLD AROUND YOU

❤ Reaping the maximum benefits of the world around you and staying connected to life outside of autism

❤ Affirmation: The Universal Connection

"Tug on anything at all and you'll find it connected to
everything else in the universe."
-John Muir

Autism is a world unto itself, isn't it? It's almost as if our autism community is a microcosm of the greater community—we've got diversity, harmony, disagreement—all the things that bind and define us a group. But certainly, we are not a group in the sense that we are isolated from the world around us. Would you like to do a great, big favor for someone you love with autism? *Do not drop out of life to get into autism!*

It's easy to learn that your child has autism and become absolutely consumed with learning everything you can about it. Learning—that's good! Too often, however, parents of children with autism stop participating in the community at large while on their quest for answers in the autism world. Not participating in community—that's bad! A primary secret to quality of life, success, and ultimately, happiness for children with autism in the mix is the level of wholeness, fulfillment, and joy that you and your child live daily. There, I've said it. Don't believe me? Consider the following undeniable truths.

In my own business over the years of teaching, training, providing therapy, and consulting exclusively in the field of autism spectrum disorders, there is a clear, defined, and recognizable pattern to my clients' successes. In virtually every case I've seen, the parents who focus on their child to the *exclusion* of focusing on their own lives do not ultimately achieve success to the same degree as parents who take care of themselves adequately. However good the intentions, I have seen this time and time again, year after year—the most well-meaning people who focus *too* hard on their child and not on themselves *burn out*. Burned out parents make bad parents. Happy, healthy parents are simply *more effective* at parenting their child, and this is especially true when autism is in the picture.

Parents of special-needs children require more self-care and self-nurturing in order to keep levels of vitality, energy, and motivation alive and working. I probably didn't need to tell you that! Yet you give yourselves less attention, less caring, less self-nurturing than parents of typical children, in a valiant attempt to give all you can to helping your child. But you parents are not *so* different, *so* separated from parents of typical children. To quote an article in my column "Inspiration: Autism," that was published a couple of years ago:

"In putting your child first, you must be ready to invest all you can afford emotionally, spiritually, and tangibly into yourself as well. Failing to nurture *your* interests, ambitions, and personality will only make you *weaker* as an advocate and healing force for your child. You cannot afford to sacrifice *so* much of yourself that, when your child needs you the most, *there is nothing left of the real you.* By caring for yourself, your ability to bring healing and light into your own child's world will soar."

Knowing this truth and sharing it makes my work—and yours—so much easier to achieve. When the goal is delivery of life improvements for a person with autism, I must insist that *every* care is taken to secure success for that child. Simply put, folks, with all the therapies, doctors, programs and consultants in the world combined, if the parents are burned out, or missing some of what *their* life's mission is, the whole formula for success becomes diluted, chaotic, fumbled, and ultimately, weakened.

It's great if you subscribe to *Autism-Asperger's Digest*—it's informative, cutting-edge, and supportive. But it's even better if you subscribe to the *Digest* and *O Magazine* or *Sports Illustrated*, taking time to brush up on what Oprah and friends can share with you on spirit, joy, and life for *you*, or how your favorite football athlete is faring these days!

It's wonderful if you go to occupational therapy to help your child develop stronger body skills. But it's *even better* if you also go to massage therapy for yourself every now and then—you've got enough stresses to justify that expense at any time! As professionals in the autism field, the good ones at least, we put so much emphasis on our passion and what we're doing for our clients, that we often forget there's more to life than professional journals, watching every TV program about autism, and taking every single two-hour long phone call as it comes from every parent. We work hard, we are exhausted trying to make that one, single impact that benefits a child for her lifetime. We want to be your hero, parents, and we want to be your child's hero. In doing so, we often find ourselves letting down our own loved ones or ourselves. It's human to do so, when a passion exists for improving the quality of life for a child with autism. But it is not the correct, natural state of being. We must recharge our spiritual batteries, our personalities, our own sense of self in order to serve you clearly.

Parents, if we are bad as professionals at taking care of ourselves, you are the *worst*! Your children matter so much to you that *you* no longer matter to you! You easily lose yourself in hours and hours of reading about autism—long gone are the days of the suspense novels you used to love. You give up your own schedule to make time for the autism schedule—drive to school at 7:00, pick up at 2:00, drive straight to the OT, stop for snacks on the way home, ABA therapist at home for an hour, then it's straight into the daily home routine—you know the drill. Multiply that by hippo therapy, speech therapy, hydrotherapy, craniosacral therapy, oral motor therapy, social skills therapy— it's enough to put *you* in therapy! You must always be working avidly to provide your child the very best of everything, because what if you slip up? What if you miss something? What if the answer is there right in front of your face and you don't see it because you are doing something that's frivolous, that's just for fun, when there is so much work to do for your child!? Who will advocate, who will help, who will support, who will drive, feed, bathe, dress, tuck in, read story, play video, find Barney doll, change sheets? Who?? *Sigh.* And then, morning comes again.

If the rhythm of your life seems to be a bit off, then I invite you to rediscover your own life. Do it for yourself. Do it for your child. Just do it! There are so many wonderful people, things, and places in this world that are waiting for you. *Your life does not stop because you're dealing with autism.* It can actually begin to take on an even greater value for you, if you will let it!

You are not dead! Yes, that's right—it's shocking, but true— you are alive! If you're not sure about this, I'm sure you can enlist the help of a medical professional who will generously agree to take your pulse free of charge and prove it to you if necessary! Unbelievably, a lot of parents with autistic children forget they are alive the minute they receive their child's diagnosis. As strange as it sounds, they actually stop doing the things they enjoy, the things that define who they *are*, and focus every single ounce of their energy on autism. I'm talking about simple, love-ly hobbies such as bike riding, reading, painting, going out to dinner with friends, jogging, yoga, the gym, writing poetry, see-ing movies at the theater *before* they come out on DVD (and Disney movies your kids want to watch don't count), buying pretty lingerie to spark some loving fun with your spouse, and more! If you think about it, it's kind of creepy, isn't it? A bunch of hobby-less, humorless shells of empty, depersonalized people walking around like zombies chasing this thing: "autism." I don't want to think about it. I just want to remind you that you *are* alive, and that *there is so very much that is unique, wonderful, and important about who you really are that your child with autism needs to see, know, and experience.* You need to see, know, and experience who you really are once again! Feel yourself come alive again. Forget about autism for awhile—it's not going any-where. It'll be right here for you when you get back from your girls' night out, your arena football game, or jet-skiing at the lake with friends for the weekend.

If you take your eyes off of autism for one minute, what's the worst that could happen? Nothing! Your child isn't going to regress because you watched a soap opera, went to get a beer with buddies, or decided to go out on your first dinner date in six months! You won't come home to find that your verbal child doesn't speak anymore, that your reading child doesn't read any-more, or that your socializing child doesn't socialize anymore. I know—it's difficult to accept this, because that is what happened to many parents when their children first started showing signs of autism. Things that were okay for the first stretch didn't carry over into the second developmental stretch. But there is no evidence that autism regresses after the onset. So breathe easy, Mom and Dad—the fear of losing more of your child can be released. It's over. It's okay now.

Why would you sit around the house depressed about autism—autism wasn't thinking about you when it entered your child's life! Don't give it all your energy. Give your *life* your energy, and share all that you can with your child. Now hurry up and put this book down so that you can go have lunch with your friends! Go on—I'll be right here when you get back!

AFFIRMATION: CONNECTING WITH THE WORLD

I am a part of the human family. I am a part of the world. I am the same person I used to be before I learned that my child has autism.

Today, I begin to nourish the person that I am. Today, I choose to live a full, rich, joyful life that goes way beyond autism!

I am connected to everyone around me! I am delighted to bring my personality, thoughts, beliefs, and support into my community. Not everything in my life has to revolve around autism! I believe that my child is more than a diagnosis—she/he is a remarkable human being, a whole child. If I believe this about my child, then surely, I must believe it about myself!

Today, I promise to do at least three very special, non-autism things for myself. If I want to do more than three special things, I will do them!

But I will not do less than three, because I must work constantly to keep myself connected to the world, and remember that we are all together in this giant, amazing universe.

I am not alone, and I will no longer act as if I am alone. I am plugged in to all that life has to offer me! I am connected with the world!

CHAPTER EIGHT

LEAD TO SUCCEED

❤ How you can change the way we view autism by raising your gentle voice of autism inspiration

❤ Affirmation: My Voice of Hope

"Be the change you wish to see in the world."
-Gandhi

You know, it's unfortunate, but not everybody in the autism world is as smart as you are! That's right—they haven't all figured out the things that you've been figuring out right here in this book, and on your own as you forge ahead on this path with your child. If you're anything like me, you are constantly thinking about ways that you can help other people live happy, productive lives (is that just me?). I think that way every day, simply because I understand that we are all connected, and that the good I bring into the life of one person can become the good she brings into the lives of many! Your experience and wisdom as collected along this autism journey is precious, unique, and valuable. You can make a choice to share your experiences with others, thereby uplifting them, inspiring them, and helping them to succeed. Doesn't that sound wonderful? It is—and it takes nothing more than a little bit of heart.

People in the autism community choose to make a monumental difference in all kinds of different ways. Lenny Schafer, father to a wonderful son with autism, started the most comprehensive email list that sends out articles about autism to masses of subscribers worldwide. Margie and Martin Truax started The Model Classroom and CADEF, the Childhood Autism Foundation, in response to their son being born with autism. And Eustacia Cutler wrote a book about what it was like being Temple Grandin's mother, *A Thorn in My Pocket*. These are great contributions to the world of autism—but you do not have to undertake a major project in order to help others. How about simply being a member of your local ASA chapter, and keeping your ears open for the sounds of new parents who are overwhelmed and in need of some hope and support? Could you write a paragraph about autism and submit it to your school or church newsletter during Autism Awareness Month? Could you answer a question on a local autism online message board about what doctor to see in your local area for help with a diagnosis? Would you attend a local charity function and splurge by buying a cool item from their silent auction? It doesn't take a lot to be an autism angel to somebody else. It just takes an open heart. You can give your own very special blend of gifts to those who need you in whatever way seems a fit for you. You don't have to do much—you don't really even have to plan it or think about it. Someday, maybe many days, the opportunity will present itself for you to do something kind or helpful in the world of autism. And because you're a part of this wide, connected world, it will feel wonderful when you choose to help out. You can put a bumper sticker on your car that shows your support for those with autism. You can offer your assistance by making a community event or program accessible to someone with autism. You can buy a copy of this book, or any book that has touched you in the world of autism, and donate it to a school or family in an area where income is an issue. The best thing to do to invite opportunities where you can help is to simply make it known that *you are here* in our autism community. Whether it's inviting a new mom to meet you for lunch—and letting her know that it's alright that her child will need to sit in her lap at the restaurant, or calling your child's teacher and letting her know that a program about Asperger's will be airing tomorrow night, you are doing your part. Don't be afraid to get in there and do something. You don't need to be a SuperParent, or one of those perfect, always involved, always made-up and coiffed moms, or one of those wealthy, donate-thousands-a-pop dads. You don't need to be an expert, you don't need to have been "through the ropes" already, and you don't need to have all the answers. You just need to care. And chances are, you already do.

One of our world's greatest sages, Gandhi, said it best: "Be the change you wish to see in the world." I'm betting that when *you* become a part of the change, you'll feel the change, better than ever.

AFFIRMATION: LEAD TO SUCCEED

My life does not exist in a vacuum. Everything that happens to me has already happened to somebody else, and will happen still again to someone else. When an opportunity presents itself, as surely it will, for me to help in the world of autism, I will rise to the occasion. Other people have helped me to reach the place I am today with understanding and acceptance for this thing called autism. I am delighted to reciprocate to the world by being a living presence to help enhance the greater changes that are yet to come for those children and adults with autism.

There are many ways to give in this world. I don't have to give specifically to the autism community, but since autism is a special part of my life, I understand the value that I may bring into the autism world.

I cannot give away that which I do not have. If I am giving in the world of autism, it means I have reached a special place of peace that I can share with others.

It is my pleasure to give from my heart to help people who are side by side with me in this autism community.

CHAPTER NINE

AUTISM AND THE DIVINE

❤ How God and spirituality can play a role in keeping your heart full and your worries light

❤ Affirmation: Feeling God

"God is a comedian playing to an audience that
is too afraid to laugh."
-Voltaire

"See God in every person, place, and thing,
and all will be well in your world."
-Louise Hay

It's perfectly okay if you're squirming as you reach this last chapter, wondering if I'm going to lose you, go into some religious rant, or otherwise disappoint you. I would be, too, if I didn't know myself! I don't believe that will happen here, and I certainly hope that's not the case, because there is no specific religious content to what I'm about to say. There's a good solid bit of spiritual observation imparted here, so if you're not into that, it's okay if you want to call it a day and close it here, no harm done and no offense taken. But I hope you don't. Whether you believe in God, or something else, or nothing else, my message in this chapter is one that ties every other chapter together (I've been told this is considered skillful and valuable when writing a book). I believe in God, and I believe that God has a tremendous sense of humor. God gave me asthma and planted me in Georgia (the allergy capital of the U.S.), dark brown curly hair when I really like red, and gave me champagne taste on a beer budget. So I'd like to approach this subject of spirituality, God, and autism from the same humorous place that I believe God came from in planning me!

You should know that, of all the resources in existence to help your child with autism, God—or the universe, or whatever you want to call it—is the only resource that nobody has taken time to write a manual, teaching text, or research study on. You can figure out how to design activity schedules for your child with autism—Woodbine House has published a book on that. You can figure out 1001 great ideas for your child with autism—Future Horizons has published a book on that. And you can read the stories of dozens of parents and professionals sharing their experiences with autism in all kinds of books—there are many published on that. Why isn't there a special book that teaches us how to use God to help navigate the world of autism? I'm not talking about a religiously-slanted book that comes from a particular Christian, Jewish, Hindu, Buddhist, Wiccan, or Snoopy-Worshipping angle. I'm not talking about anybody trying to put a brand name on God's input here, using their spiritual text as a final source, or claiming it for their religious party.

If you'll allow me, I'll like to share my humble attempt at giving you a sense of how to use God in your autism intervention. Although I'm not a preacher, a rabbi, or a spiritual warrior, I do feel qualified to teach you about God and autism—because I believe I know both of them very well. After all, God created me, so surely I've picked up some divine qualities that way! And as for knowing autism—well, you've read my book so far, and the fact that you've kept on going is hopeful!

You can call it whatever your heart resonates with—science, the Universe, energy, nature, or God. I choose to call "it" God, but you're free to substitute your own language of choice to make this chapter suitable for you. I believe that God is absolutely kind, and would want you to know these things without wondering anymore. So if I may, I'd like to act as a Divine Ambassador of sorts, and deliver the thoughts that I think God would like you to have in your autism intervention repertoire, starting today.

I Created Your Child With Autism Because I Love You— And Your Child—So Much. That's the reason, that's the purpose, and that's it. You might think there's no way that it's that simple, but the truth is, there's no way that it's any more complicated. Everything I do for you is out of love, and that's my only motivation, ever. Autism is not a punishment, a mistake, or a curse. It is a part of human existence that, like every other aspect of who you are, is a blessing, and a gift. Autism is your opportunity to see the things that reside within you that you wish could be different—and to change them. As human beings, don't you often wish that you had more opportunities to give to others, to act with meaning and purpose, and to work towards some great cause? Then I have given you children with autism, and so you are blessed with opportunities for all of these, because they need you!

Often, do you not wish that you could simply be yourself in front of others, with all of your quirky unique behaviors and private, silly habits? Then I have given you children with autism—learn from them! They are content with who they are, and they need not conform or find the acceptance of others to love themselves. Learn from them! Do you have a passion for something—maybe writing, maybe gardening, maybe protecting abused children, maybe building model trains, maybe helping endangered animals—but ignore your passion because you are too busy working hard and earning income? Look to your children with autism—see how they light up and thrive with focus on their passions! They throw their hearts and minds into the causes that they care for, and you can do this, too! Have you been dealing with relationships that are unfulfilling, or have you remained connected to people who do not truly reflect the wonderful, kind of person that you are? Then watch how your children with autism handle relationships. They interact with others when it is meaningful, valuable, and rewarding to them—not to please anyone else! In return, they give uniquely of themselves in a way that I am sure you understand. Rather than throw the words "I love you" around, or constantly engage in symbolic rituals that stand for love, they simply feel overwhelmed with love for you at all times inside! That love is so powerful that they do not feel they need to tell you!

You Can Create A Fulfilling Experience With Your Child. If your child is not currently at a stage of development or ability where she/he can meet your emotional needs as a parent, then you can return to me through the workings of your creative heart, and I will help you! To do this, simply close your eyes and imagine yourself in any beautiful place that you can love—a field with a rustic brown barn, a sandy beach with a lighthouse, a garden filled with roses that leads to a stone cottage. As you take steps through the natural environment, you get closer and closer to the building in sight. As you approach the building, you notice that your child is there, inside, waiting with a warm smile for you! You open the doors to the building, and hear them swing open with a creak in the hinges. You enter the building, and see your child waiting in the center of the room! Here, together, you may ask your child anything! You may ask your child about feelings, thoughts, experiences—anything you'd like to know! In this place, your child is free of the differences that make it difficult for you to converse freely at home. In this place, your child can speak freely, just as you can. Take your time, my dear one, and ask your child all the questions within your loving heart—and then listen one by one as they are answered! When you have completed your special visit, you may kiss your child, say a temporary goodbye, and walk slowly out of the building, and back through the outdoors to your starting point. Here, I will return you to your regular life, and you are free to incorporate what you have learned and experienced with your child into your daily life! Anytime you feel like having another special visit with your child, simply call upon Me, and I will gladly escort you back to your very special meeting place!

I Will Always Come When You Call. The truth is, I am never absent from your side, so you may rest assured knowing that I am always right there with you. In the carpool line when you are in a hurry to get to speech therapy, I am there with you. At the grocery store when your child frets over wanting a cereal that you will not buy, I am there with you. And when you simply need a moment alone to recharge, I am there with you! But since it is sometimes hard for you humans to remember that I am always there, perhaps it will help you to simply remember that I will gladly come to your side anytime that you call upon me. I am not too busy, and nothing else is more important. I am here for you whenever you need me, for whatever reasons you may need me, and in any way that you need me.

Trust Your Feelings. When you get feelings about what choices to make for your child's autism intervention, you should trust them. I am with you during these times, and I am often behind the feelings that you have! Sometimes, these "feelings" are really just quiet guidance that I am sharing with you. You can trust them!

I Do Not Work Alone. It may brighten your spirits to learn that there are many special divinely inspired helpers who are with you along your autism journey! Sometimes you may feel the presence of the Autism Angel herself, who has been a great inspiration for Jennifer in writing this book, and in all the work that she does. Likewise, the Autism Angel may be an inspiration to you. There are other individuals who are in your life to help as well. Have you been blessed with a wonderful teacher, a talented therapist, a supportive spouse? All of these people—and many more—are with you to help me assist you on your autism journey! Sometimes, people will emerge from nowhere to help, only to disappear the next week—and yet they did their divinely inspired job to reach you somehow! Recognize that there are many people in your life now—and soon to enter it—who are working with Me to help you. Doesn't that feel wonderful?

It Is Always Okay. Nothing that happens in your child's life with autism will be catastrophic. It is always okay. There is nothing happening to your child that I am not watching, and there is nothing happening to you that I am not watching. You are always loved, cherished, and safe. If your child falls, then the next step will be getting up. If your child gets hurt, then the next step will be healing. If your child suffers, then the next step will be experiencing peace. What seems like pain is never really lasting. It is only a brief, temporary step along the journey that autism has blessed you with.

You Can Remember Me. Other people—even religious people—may forget Me, or even forget My true loving nature. This is okay. Some people are afraid of how their lives will change if they believe that I only feel love for them. This is sometimes true about places where religious people congregate, and at other times, this is not true about those places. Know that if you can remember me, then it makes no difference where you remember me. I enter every house, and I pay no regard to the name of the house, how many people are in the house, or what the people are saying inside the house. If you go to a church to talk to me, I will welcome you. If you find that a church or synagogue or other house will not welcome your child, I will welcome you. It is not important that a house makes you feel welcome, it is important that you make me welcome in your house. The rest will follow, this I promise! Your prayers can be heard from everywhere!

You Must Laugh. Autism is not meant to be a serious burden, but a lighthearted blessing in your life! Do not forget to give the gift of togetherness through laughter to your child. Since it is true that I will never give you more than you can handle, why are you so serious? You can be laughing with delight instead, knowing that you are as strong and capable as I am! You must laugh when you understand that your child with autism is also as strong and capable as I am! Do you understand how and in what ways? It does not matter if you understand—you must simply know it to be true, and laugh! Nothing brings the angels to you faster than the sound of your heartfelt laughter!

You Are Amongst Angels. Even as you know that I do not work alone, you will at times forget how very supported you are. You should know that there are scores of angels at your side daily, and the sole purpose of their presence is to constantly support you! These angels are not just here because of autism, but because of every piece of who you are. They love you, just as I do, and they help guide you. These angels can "run spiritual errands" for you, if you will just take a moment to delegate to them! Do you need greater financial abundance to help pay for a special therapy? Ask an angel to go find extra funding for you! Do you want a quiet vacation but feel unsure of when vacation time will come? Ask an angel to bring it forth for you! Do you need some rest and quiet time to reflect upon your own life? Ask an angel to create this time for you! You may ask an angel any-thing—from help with rekindling romance in your marriage, to alleviating the strain between family members due to disagree-ments about how to address your child's autism. The angels who are with you are there solely to help you, so let them!

There Is No Limit To My Love. Nothing you have ever done, whether regarding autism, or your own life, or anything else, has ever been unacceptable to me. You cannot feel a single drop of guilt, remorse, or responsibility for your child's autism or for the way that you have handled it up to this point. Everything that you have done has been perfect. Everything that you will do will be perfect. For any act that is followed by learning later is truly perfect, regardless of the immediate result. And for every perfect gesture you have made, and every loving lesson you have so will-ingly and openly learned, I love you with no limit. I will always love you. And that is what I needed you to know.

Today, my wish for you is that you find all the wisdom in these words. Whether you embrace them as sentiments from a believer in God, or the creation of a loving person who cares about her readers, I hope that they have touched you. All the autism intervention in the world cannot replace the value of a confident, loving, and caring parent or teacher who feels fully supported in this work. So I have taught you what I know, and now, in this final chapter, I have also shared what I believe. If something in this book has brought knowledge or happiness or peace into your perspective on autism, then I have met my goal. My goal, as you know, is to improve the quality of life for individuals with autism, one heart at a time. Which heart is your child's? I hope that I have reached it.

Which heart is yours? I hope that I have filled it.

And if I have, I ask for only one thing in return—that you take a moment of your life, a deep breath, and go ahead and make a goal of your own. What is your goal, then? Is it to improve your child's life? To help those with autism? To build a beautiful garden? To touch the stars with your beautiful written stories? I ask that you make a goal for yourself, and devote a portion of your life to meeting it. Nothing is more fulfilling to me than helping other people meet their goals. This philosophy certainly helps me in IEP meetings and in classrooms with children who have autism. But it also extends to others—to men, women, parents, grandparents—whom I am blessed to come in contact with through their lovable, remarkable children. Your child has brought me to your fingertips. Perhaps your child, in loving thanks for the hard work that you do, is here in part to help you remember your own passions and goals.

Figure them out. Make a plan to meet those goals. And write to me to tell me about it!

Teachers, parents, professionals, and friends, I applaud you for your work in the field of autism. Now go—do something beautiful for yourselves!

With Love, Light, and Laughter,

Jennifer

AFFIRMATION: SPIRITUALITY AND AUTISM

It surprised me at first to read about spirituality and autism together. The world does not often place spiritual value on everyday things. Yet here I am, affirming my own truths to a higher power, and I realize—autism is connected to God and spirituality!

There is nothing that is separate from anything else. We are all connected, including God, me, and my child with autism. When I stop to remember this, I feel happier, safer, more at ease in the world of autism. It's as if a weight has been lifted off my shoulders, and off my child's shoulders. It's true—I do not have to worry. There is a kind of Divine support that is a part of my life.

I accept the blessings of all the kindness, love, and joy in this world. I accept that these blessings can play a role in my child's life with autism! And I believe firmly that, no matter what happens in my life, I am supported by a special network of help that will not give me any more than I can handle.

Knowing that I am not alone is the perfect way to soothe my spirit.

EPILOGUE

True universal wisdom is never "new." It is timeless. Five wise men summarized the message of *The Heart Of Autism* long before the book was ever written.

The first was Johann Wolfgang von Goethe. He said:

"Treat people as if they were what they ought to be, and you help them to become what they are capable of being."

Imagine this applied in the world of autism. It evokes imagery of a world where people with autism are treated as bright, intelligent, loving, and capable human beings. How would they respond to such treatment? What joys, achievements, and fulfillment would be certain for every person with autism dwelling in his or her heart if only we would first invest our beliefs and confidences in them? This book asks you to explore it now. It would be a world where teachers were not judged as skimming on their responsibilities, being undereducated or ill-equipped in their fields, or lacking the warmth and passion to reach every child—yes, *every* child. Instead, teachers would be treated like gold, like angelic bridges between hopes and realities for every student. They would not hide from their power, but shine brighter in it. They would not shy away from the responsibilities that come with teaching, but rather, be fueled by them. This book asks you to explore this now. And then there are the parents. No longer would anyone view parents as the force that holds their children with autism back, the incapable influence that unravels what is worked towards so tirelessly in the classroom, the misguided voice of desperation that throws

153

progress off track, or the indifferent bystander who waits for others to "undo" the autism in their child's life. Instead, parents would be treated with irrepressible reverence, absolute support, and unconditional love akin to the truth that shines forth from them for their children. They would be celebrated and thanked and embraced daily at every corner. They would be praised for courageously and selflessly accepting the world's only true full-time job, and for doing it with nearly seamless energy, enthusiasm, and positive results at hand. This is what my book is about. This is the message. We can all rise to the occasion, if only we will choose to treat each other with the loving kindness, respect, and dignity that each one of us is absolutely, positively, and universally worth. Treat others this way. Treat yourself this way.

The second gentleman was James Crook, who said:

"The man who wants to lead the orchestra must turn his back on the crowd."

In the end, it will not matter what other people have done for their children with autism. It will only matter what you have done for your child with autism. People in this world often make poor decisions for good reasons, and good decisions for poor reasons. It's only human, and you can't measure your actions by theirs, for fear of doing more of the same. Forget about what others are doing. James Crook knew that. Your mother knew that. And you and I both know it now. This book reminds you of your own wisdom. Do what is right for your child. Don't follow the trends. Follow what makes sense, and shows real, measurable results in your child's daily progress. To do this, you may need to turn your back on the crowd—but this book reminds you that you aren't here to view or follow the autism crowd. You're here to lead your child's heart in a very heavenly symphony that only you can conduct. Lead your child's orchestra of intervention now. Don't focus on the others. Let them watch you, and learn. Your child will thank you, and your legacy in song will be more beautiful than you've ever imagined.

The third wise man was the talented Ernest Hemingway. He said:

"Never mistake motion for action."

Stop the motion and think about this for just a moment. In the world of autism education and intervention, are you simply moving around, or are you boldly taking action? Moving in circles will eventually—and sometimes heartbreakingly—take you back to your starting point. Only *forward* movement can be judged as true action. Are you talking about, researching, and exploring the source of your child's autism, running yourself around in dizzying circles but getting nowhere? Are you permanently going through the motions of blame, of anger, of unsettled disgust or the rise and fall of emotions over a potential cause or a potential cure or a potential dream that is lost and found, or found and lost? Stop spinning your wheels—you deserve more, and your child's life requires more. Instead, are you seeing progress of some kind? Are you leaving the negative thoughts and emotions behind that were yours from years, months, weeks, even days ago and rapidly welcoming their positive, forward-driven replacements? There is no time for simple motion. You need to respond to autism with action. It is not action to talk about the same angry thought over and over and over again. It is not action to hit the "pause" button on responsible, thorough, and supportive intervention while you stop to explore possible sources of this autism and its manifestations. You may explore, but you must not confuse that motion with true action. Give your students 100% each day in class, refreshed and new. Give your child access to the best therapies, programs, and interventions because they do make a difference. Give yourself as parents a quality of life that is rich, full, and rewarding independent of autism and all that goes with it. Make this a quality of life that does not diminish in an effort to give your child everything— that's a surefire motion that lands you back at the starting line every time. Give your child all you can. Give your students all you can. Do so not just in concept with words, but back your words with actions. Our first wise man, Goethe, compliments Hemingway's sentiment, saying, *"To think is easy. To act is difficult. To act as one thinks is the most difficult."* This book serves to remind you of this.

The fourth wise sage is Albert Einstein. Einstein said:

"In the midst of difficulty lies opportunity."

So you've been dealt a hand that includes autism for you or someone you love. It is an indisputably difficult hand to play in the game of life. Albert Einstein would have us focus not on the obvious difficulty, but on the subtle reality of opportunity hidden within the presence of autism. There are triumphs to cherish that no one else will ever know. There are opportunities for true growth, not just for someone with autism. They are opportunities for growth in *you*. You can become a student's greatest teacher. You can inspire a child's greatest achievements. You can learn to intercept the seemingly horrid aches and pains of your own life, and hold the bright candle of autism to them to put it all into perspective. False obstacles and treacherous superficial details will fall away from your life, while you watch as others without autism near them grapple over mundane, inconsequential things that you are freed from focusing on because you have been given the opportunity to know what really matters. It could always be better, and for some other mother, father, teacher, therapist, or person with autism, it undoubtedly is. But it could always be worse, and for some other mother, father, teacher, therapist, or person with autism, it undoubtedly is. Human beings are built to endure, to persist, and to ultimately succeed in attaining joy. Circumstance—however dreary—cannot derail human nature. Autism cannot derail human nature. You were designed with a great capacity to demonstrate resilience in the face of challenge. You were designed to experience as much joy and love as the human heart can hold, which to this day remains immeasurable. Bounce back from a diagnosis of autism. Be resilient. Give way to your inspiring human nature, to your sparkling, shining, God-given soul. You will not only survive this difficulty, but you will benefit from it with endless opportunities for more than you ever dreamed of. So will your student. So will your child. Remember that.

Gandhi is our fifth and final sage, who gave us the following wisdom:

"I offer you peace. I offer you love. I offer you friendship. I see your beauty. I hear your need. I feel your feelings. My wisdom flows from the Highest Source. I salute that Source in you. Let us work together for unity and love."

This is what *The Heart Of Autism* is meant to teach us all. When we treat each other and view each other with these kinds of loving eyes, then our autism world will truly begin to reflect the kind of peace, unity, and love that every one of us is worthy of. And so, my closing thought to you is this:

My dear reader in the world of autism, I offer you peace. I offer you love. I see your beauty. I hear your need. I feel your feelings. My wisdom flows from the Highest Source. I salute that Source in you. Let us work together for unity and love.

Let us work together to improve the quality of life for individuals with autism, one heart at a time. It is the best work on earth, and it belongs to you and me.

Jennifer

ABOUT THE AUTHOR

Jennifer Abeles is better known throughout the worldwide autism community as the Autism Angel. She has served autistic individuals of all ages and abilities in nearly every capacity imaginable. Her no-nonsense, positive, and effective approach to autism intervention combined with her inspiring attitude has made her one of the most sought after speakers, trainers, and consultants in the field of autism today.

Jennifer is the founder and Executive Director of the Autism Angel Center, the non-profit autism resource center providing highly specialized direct service programs, resources, and professional and parent trainings. The Center's signature programs are the Autism Angel Program—the full time, year round, comprehensive private early intervention classroom providing individualized one-on-one, small group, and inclusion learning, and Social Butterflies—inclusive social skills groups serving children ages three and up through art, music, silly snack, and fun movement activities. The programs are based on reputable best practices in autism intervention and incorporate the unique interests, personalities, and needs of each participating child. With her hands-on direct and personal role, Jennifer brings her own beloved blend of inspiration and effective strategizing to the table for the children served in both programs.

Jennifer continues to hold the appreciation, respect, and admiration of professionals internationally, training colleagues and educators with backgrounds from paraprofessionals to Ph.D's in best practices for addressing individuals with autism.

Her goal is to improve the quality of life for individuals with autism, one heart at a time.

The Autism Angel currently makes her home in beautiful, vibrant Athens, Georgia, where, aside from running the Autism Angel Center and working with children, she delights in reading, making whimsical arts and crafts for fun, collecting fairies, dragonflies, butterflies, and angels, spending time in nature and traveling, remembering to play and laugh, and writing on many topics ranging from autism to political ethics, angels, the human spirit, philosophy and "anything that comes to mind and heart that might help inspire someone, empower someone, or make someone think." She lives with her wonderful husband Mark, who is a technology executive, their three dogs—Oscar, Lexi, and Harvey—and a little colony of happy dustbunnies presently residing under their comfy bed.

Visit the Autism Angel's Official Website:

www.theautismangel.org

Contact the Autism Angel:

Jennifer@theautismangel.org

THE AUTISM ANGEL
PENDANT PROJECT

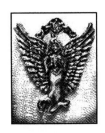

Wear it to show that you believe in someone with autism.
Wear it to support and honor someone with autism.
Wear it because you love someone with autism.

Feel the positive, uplifting support and inspiration of the Autism Angel every time you wear the pendant near to your heart. 100% of all profits from the sale of every pendant go to support and develop autism programs, resources, scholarships, and intervention sponsored by the Autism Angel Center in Northeast Georgia.

The Autism Angel Pendant is not a mass-produced generic fundraising item! Each pendant is a collector's item, handmade by jewelry artisan Kirk "Merlin" McLaren in the finest quality pure sterling silver. The back of each pendant bears the insignia mark of the Autism Angel (her signature "autism" heart with wings) and is signed and numbered by the artist. Each comes with a numbered certificate of authenticity that is personally hand-signed (not photocopied) by Jennifer Abeles and Kirk McLaren.

$45 for the sterling silver pendant,

$56 for the sterling silver and gemstone pendant.

Shipping and handling is $2 for the first pendant. Additional pendants shipped within the same order are mailed without additional shipping charges.

Please note that whenever possible, your pendant will be shipped within 2-3 business days. Because each individual pendant is handcrafted, it may take 4-6 weeks for your pendant to be shipped in the event that it is not available at the time your order is received. If you require your order to reach you earlier than this, please email us before placing your order. Order inquiries can be sent to pendant@theautismangel.org.

Printed in the United States
129362LV00004B/16/A